Pharmocracy II

Pharmocracy II

*How Corrupt Deals and Misguided Medical
Regulations Are Bankrupting America—
and What to Do About It*

William Faloon

Co-founder of the
Life Extension Foundation Buyers Club

DISCLAIMER

Ideas and information in this book are based upon the experience and training of the author and the scientific information currently available. The suggestions in this book are definitely not meant to be a substitute for careful medical evaluation and treatment by a qualified, licensed health professional. The author and publisher do not recommend changing or adding medication or supplements without consulting your personal physician. They specifically disclaim any liability arising directly or indirectly from the use of this book.

Axios Press
PO Box 457
Edinburg, VA 22824
888.542.9467   info@axiosinstitute.org

Library of Congress Cataloging-in-Publication Data

Names: Faloon, William, author.
Title: Pharmocracy II : how corrupt deals and misguided medical regulations are bankrupting America and what to do about it / William Faloon.
Other titles: Pharmocracy 2 | Pharmocracy two
Description: Edinburg, VA : Axios, [2017] | Includes bibliographical references and index. |
Identifiers: LCCN 2017024252 (print) | LCCN 2017025051 (ebook) | ISBN 9781604191226 () | ISBN 9781604191219 (hardcover)
Subjects: | MESH: United States. Food and Drug Administration. | Drug Industry--economics | Fees, Pharmaceutical | Health Policy--economics | Government Agencies | Government Regulation | United States
Classification: LCC HD9665.5 (ebook) | LCC HD9665.5 (print) | NLM QV 736 AA1 | DDC 338.4/76151--dc23
LC record available at https://lccn.loc.gov/2017024252

Contents

Preface

HEALTHCARE IS BANKRUPTING the United States.

Medical costs have escalated to a level that individuals, businesses, and debt-laden governments can no longer afford to pay.

There is a real-world solution.

Congress can create legislation that will allow free-market forces to drive down sick-care costs, better enable disease prevention, and rapidly perfect curative therapies.

This book provides factual documentation on how broken the US healthcare system is today. It is over 300 pages long because there are at least that many reasons why healthcare costs far more than it should.

Until now, no one has identified and amalgamated the plethora of illogical regulations that directly cause healthcare to be so overpriced.

While this book attacks FDA corruption and ineptitude, Congress is the body of government that provides the FDA with enabling laws that ultimately result in needless human suffering and death—while the nation descends into financial ruination.

Implementing free-market approaches can spare Medicare and Medicaid from insolvency, while significantly improving the health and productivity of the American public.

Pharmocracy II provides an irrefutable and rational basis to remove the suffocating compulsory aspect of healthcare regulation and allow free-market forces to compete against government-sanctioned medicine.

This book documents how the free market can provide superior healthcare at far lower prices while better protecting consumers.

Disregard of the obvious problems revealed in this book will condemn the United States to a downward economic spiral with little improvement in healthy human longevity.

—William Faloon

Introduction

A FIERCE DEBATE IS RAGING as to who will pay for this nation's skyrocketing "sick-care" costs.

Private companies have scaled back sharply on the healthcare coverage they used to provide.[1,2] Employees now pay an increasing percentage of their medical insurance premiums, along with higher deductibles, co-pays, and no-pays (i.e., exclusions). Many businesses provide their employees with no health coverage.

Based on the median income in the United States, the typical family cannot come close to paying the staggering cost of healthcare themselves.

It seems rather odd, but since neither the private business sector nor individuals can afford today's sick-care costs, the burden is increasingly being borne by the sector least able to pay, i.e., heavily indebted local, state, and federal governments.

Even those covered by government insurance (such as municipal employees and Medicare recipients) are facing higher medical insurance premiums.

The federal government is already saddled with a huge unfunded Medicare liability. No one has figured out where the money will come from to cover these future health-care costs.

To put Medicare alone into context, in year 2015, the unfunded liability stood at $27 trillion to $43.5 trillion, depending on which federal agency projection you look at.[3] Yet total federal tax revenue taken in annually (which includes Medicare premiums) is only around $3.2 trillion.[4]

President Obama stated in 2010 that we are approaching a point where government will have to spend more money on Medicare than on every other federal program combined![5,6] In the ensuing seven years, however, nothing has been done by any politician to address the massive unfunded healthcare liability the United States (and other nations) must contend with.

The Medicare unfunded liability does not count the escalating costs of Medicaid (sick-care coverage for the poor) that are shared by federal and state governments. Medicaid is funded with current tax revenue and newly issued debt, but its spiraling growth has created a new multi-trillion dollar unfunded liability, and no one knows where the money will come from to pay it.[7]

Bernard Madoff was sentenced to 150 years in prison because he took investors' money and diverted it to other purposes. The federal government forced Americans to pay Medicare premiums their entire lives. Instead of those premiums being placed in a reserve fund for future use, they were squandered on whatever was most politically expedient at the time, which included overpaying—with tax dollars—those with the right political connections.

While Madoff will spend the rest of his life incarcerated, no one talks about bringing civil or criminal charges against those responsible for what may be the largest Ponzi scheme in the history of the human race: Medicare, with its >$27 trillion of unfunded liabilities.

Like the federal government, many local and state governments have also operated a Ponzi scheme of unfunded pension and healthcare liabilities they cannot pay.[8] State and local governments long ago promised their employees free or heavily subsidized healthcare for life. Skyrocketing sick-care costs, combined with increases in human longevity, have made it impossible for these promised healthcare benefits to be fulfilled under today's over-regulated environment that causes medicine to exponentially cost more than it should.

Since the federal government is mathematically insolvent, it seems ludicrous to assume that exorbitant sick-care costs can be resolved by any level of government.

While politicians point fingers over who should pay America's medical bills, please remember that there is a real-world solution.

Healthcare in the United States is so tightly regulated that it in many ways resembles the inefficiencies of Maoist China, where the economy suffocated for decades due to erratic and illogical governmental decrees. As China lifted its regulatory stranglehold, prosperity flourished.

It's time for US leaders to follow China's example and stop over-regulating medicine!

WE HAVE BEEN DECEIVED BY BIG PHARMA

Americans have paid outlandish prices for prescription drugs, believing that pharmaceutical profits would fund research leading to medical breakthroughs. The problem is that very few real-world discoveries have manifested. One can point to some treatments that prolong patient survival, but these are offset by lethal side effects inflicted by fraudulently approved therapies.[9-11] The fact is that few real cures have occurred, despite Americans spending more healthcare dollars than anyone else.

Examples of cures are antibiotics and vaccines that eradicated diseases. These were developed long before today's regulatory stranglehold ended these kinds of breakthrough innovations.

Since the first *Pharmocracy* was written, several pharmaceuticals have been developed that "cure" most cases of hepatitis C. While these drugs represent a major biomedical advance, their outrageous price (such as $1,000 per pill for the drug Solvaldi®) is beyond rational affordability.

Major strides have been made against chronic myeloid leukemia, but once again, drug prices exceeding $100,000 per year for the lifetime of each patient has led oncology groups to state that these costs are "unsustainable."[12,13]

Unregulated medicine continues to make considerable strides. The majority of the population, however, does not know about these approaches. Vested financial interests have spent billions to ensure that the media, politicians, and bureaucrats continue suppressing more effective and less expensive ways to prevent and treat degenerative illnesses.

Americans have been deceived by those who associate regulations with beneficial outcomes. As it relates to medical progress, relatively little has occurred for the lethal diseases impacting aging Americans. The abysmal track record of conventional medicine is a direct reflection of the "regulatory burden" that stifles development of novel and less expensive therapies.[14]

Few Americans understand that the underlying purpose of any given regulation is to provide a government-protected advantage to the group favoring that regulation. It's not about how a regulation will protect the public, but instead a matter of how can it "financially benefit a special interest."[15]

An oft-cited example is a petition the drug maker Wyeth filed with the FDA asking that a natural human form of estrogen called estriol be banned.[16] The female hormone drugs Wyeth sold (Premarin® and PremPro®) had been shown to produce side effects.[17–26] Instead of spending research dollars to come up with safer forms of estrogen (such as combining natural estrogens with indole-3-carbinol and natural progesterone),[27–33] it was much cheaper to persuade political hacks at the FDA to outlaw the competition (i.e., bioidentical estriol hormone compounds).[34]

Pharmaceutical companies have spent enormous amounts of money persuading the FDA to reclassify nutrients like pyridoxamine into prescription drugs so they can monopolize them for their own economic benefit.[35] Pyridoxamine is a form of vitamin B6 that reduces the formation of advance glycation end products.[36] It was sold as a dietary supplement for years before the FDA mandated it be removed (in 2009) because a pharmaceutical company wanted to have pyridoxamine approved as a "drug" to treat kidney disease.

Interestingly, as this book was being updated in 2017, the pyridoxamine "drug" remains bogged down in the expensive and cumbersome "approval" process. That means no American can derive its potential life-saving benefit at any price.

The FDA took away what was a low-cost dietary supplement to benefit a drug company. This provided one company with a monopoly to investigate and possibly market this non-patented version of vitamin B6 (pyridoxamine). The company owning the monopoly (courtesy of the FDA) now struggles to cover the enormous costs of having it "approved" by the same federal agency.[37]

If it were not for aggressive letter-writing campaigns by consumers to Congress, most dietary supplements would now be expensive prescription drugs, or not available at all.

FDA—FAILURE, DECEPTION, ABUSE

In 2010, I finished a 498-page book called *FDA: Failure, Deception, Abuse,* which exposed how over-regulation has destroyed citizens' health and this nation's finances.

One year later, I put together the first *Pharmocracy* book to expose more atrocities committed by out-of-control politicians and bureaucrats against our health and pocketbooks.

This book, *Pharmocracy II*, provides startling updates to a medical cost crisis that is exploding out of control.

The magnitude of the artificially inflated drug costs are beyond obscene. As I was finalizing this book, the media was focusing on a generic drug used to save the lives of children who suffer acute allergic food allergies.

The name of the drug is EpiPen®, and its cost has risen 550% since year 2007.[38] There is nothing unique about the active ingredient (epinephrine) in this injectable that parents carry to save their child's life. The maker nonetheless enjoys a virtual monopoly based on effective lobbying, aggressive legal defense against competitors, and the high costs of getting the FDA to approve competing versions of the identical drug.

The retail price for a pack of two EpiGen® pens is $608 (up from $94 in 2007).[39] Many parents cannot afford this outlandish price and risk their children slowly suffocating to death if an acute allergic reaction occurs.

In case you're wondering what it costs to make this drug, experts are quoted as stating the epinephrine put into a similar auto injector can be made for $3–$7.[40] With sterile quality control, this drug could be profitably sold for less than $100—if it were not for the power Congress bestows on the FDA to pick and choose who gets to make it.

In response to media backlash, the maker of the EpiPen® promised to make a generic version that costs only $300 . . . which is still as much as one hundred times more than what it costs to make.[41]

The $300 price for a drug that may be needed multiple times each year is still unaffordable by many parents whose deductibles are over $4,000 each year.

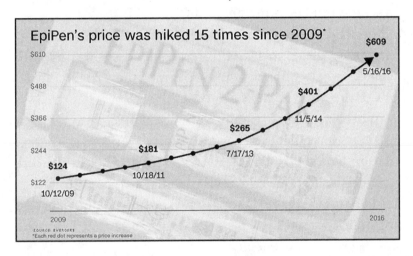

A few months after the EpiPen® disclosures, a drug used by migraine suffers shot up to $728 for nine tablets.[42] The active ingredients in this drug, called Treximet®, are generics (sumatriptan and naproxen) that long ago came off patent. If purchased separately, these same two drugs would cost consumers around $19. By combining them, the pharmaceutical company can reap in huge profits from taxpayer-funded programs like Medicare and Medicaid.

To provide an idea of how much profit there is with Treximet®, the company offers to sell it directly to hardship cases for only $20 as opposed to the $728 price that many consumers are faced with at the pharmacy counter. The company still makes a profit based on cost of product on $20 direct sales.

In this Orwellian tragedy, the annual cost of "regulated" drugs can amount to thousands of dollars whereas the same drugs in a "free market" environment would plummet considerably.

WHY CONGRESS DOES NOT ACT

Imagine a member of Congress introducing a bill repealing this kind of FDA-protected monopoly.

The pharmaceutical industry would spend whatever amount of money needed to keep this law from being enacted, and would heavily finance whoever ran against this member of Congress in the next election.

In other words, it would be political suicide to attempt to allow unregulated drugs to be sold, even though deregulation would go a long way to solving today's healthcare cost crisis. That's why consumers have to band together to demand Congress ignore pharmaceutical lobbyists and introduce emergency legislation that repeal today's absurd over-regulation of medicine.

The title of this book is *Pharmocracy II*, but I contemplated the original title as *Regulation Breeds Corruption*. The reason I considered that title is that egregious pharmaceutical company profits are protected by regulations. These vested interests will go to any corrupt length to ensure these regulations are perpetuated, no matter how inane they are.[43–45]

The word "corruption" is often interpreted as meaning something illegal. The word corruption, however, can be defined as immoral behavior, an example of which is the exploitation of a position of power for personal gain. When it comes to campaign contributions, lobbying, and offering congressional staff generous employment after they retire, these are not overtly illegal acts.[46] They routinely happen, which means this kind of devastating corruption has been institutionalized and must now be eliminated.

HOW REGULATED COSTS ADD UP

Institutionalized corruption artificially inflates the cost of virtually every healthcare service.

When one considers there are thousands of medical-related products and services that are artificially inflated by senseless regulations, it becomes clear that radical change is required to avoid an economic meltdown.

In dealing with runaway healthcare costs, a solution is to make certain drugs like statins available without the necessity of a doctor's visit. There are now companies that employ physicians to review blood tests over the phone and prescribe certain medications, but the FDA and state licensing boards are a constant threat to their existence.[47]

Corrupt regulations ensure that efficiencies that would slash healthcare costs never see the light of day.

SIMPLE SOLUTION TO AVERT ECONOMIC RUINATION

The Life Extension Foundation® initiated a petition drive back in the 1980s to allow individual Americans to "opt out" of the FDA's regulatory umbrella. Our rationale was that this would provide consumers with more advanced treatments at lower prices.

Hundreds of enlightened Life Extension Foundation® members petitioned the FDA demanding liberation from its regulatory stranglehold. The public, Congress, and the media were apathetic at that time.

The FDA was far from lethargic. They responded to our petition analogous to an angry hornet's nest (and how dictators respond to dissidents). The notion that we dared challenge the FDA's absolute authority resulted in years of legal battles where the FDA did everything in its power to try to destroy the Life Extension Foundation® (and put me in jail).[48]

Fast-forward to today. The political climate has changed. The healthcare cost crisis we long ago predicted has evolved into a harsh reality no one can ignore. It is mathematically impossible to solve it by forcing one group to pay regulated medicine's corruptly inflated costs. The only salvation is the free-market reforms that the Life Extension Foundation® long ago drafted.

Our proposal is quite simple. Change the laws to allow good-manufacturing practice-certified (GMP) manufacturing facilities to produce generic prescription drugs that do not undergo the excessive regulatory hurdles that force consumers to pay egregiously inflated prices.

To alert consumers when they are getting a generic that is not as heavily regulated as it is currently, the law would mandate that the label of these less-regulated generic drugs clearly state:

> This is not an FDA-approved manufactured generic drug and may be ineffective and potentially dangerous. This drug is not manufactured under the same standards required for an FDA-approved generic drug. Purchase this drug at your own risk.

By allowing the sale of these less costly generics, consumers will have a choice as to which companies they choose to trust.

Equally important among our proposals is one that allows consumers to be told about the off-label benefits of prescription drugs. An example is the extensive body of evidence that metformin may help prevent—not simply treat—type 2 diabetes,[49,50] and that metformin may also prevent and help treat certain cancers.[51–62]

A concern critics raise about this free-market solution is safety. Who will protect consumers from poorly made generic drugs, they ask?

First of all, the manufacturers of these drugs would be subject to the same regulation as GMP-certified over-the-counter drug and dietary supplement makers. FDA inspectors will visit facilities, take sample products, and assay them to ensure the potency of active ingredients, dissolution, etc. Manufacturers that fail to make products that meet the label's claims would face civil and criminal penalties.

Secondly, there is no incentive not to provide the full potency of active ingredients in these less-regulated generic drugs. The price of the active ingredient makes up such a small percentage of the overall cost that a manufacturer would be idiotic to scrimp on potency.[63]

Companies that foolishly make inferior generics will be viciously exposed by the media, along with the FDA, consumer protection groups, and even prescribing physicians who will be suspicious if a drug is not working as it is supposed to. (Just imagine how easy it would be to spot a bogus generic statin that did not reduce cholesterol?)

Companies producing inferior products will be quickly driven from the marketplace as consumers who choose to purchase these lower-cost generics will seek out laboratories that have reputations for making flawless products.

Substandard companies would not only be castigated in the public's eye, but also face civil litigation from customers who bought the defective generics. When one considers that GMP-certified manufacturing plants can cost hundreds of millions of dollars to set up, a company would guarantee itself future insolvency if it failed to produce generic drugs that met minimum standards.

PHARMACEUTICAL COMPANY PROPAGANDA

No matter how many facts show that free-market generic drugs will be safe, there are alarmists who believe that even if one person might suffer a serious adverse event because of a lower-cost generic drug, the law should not be amended to allow the sale of these less-regulated products.

What few understand is that enabling lower-cost drugs to be sold might reduce the number of poorly made drugs. The reason is that prescription drug counterfeiting remains a major issue.[64] Drugs are counterfeited because they are so expensive. In the free-market environment we espouse, a month's supply of a popular cholesterol-lowering drug like simvastatin would sell for less than $3.00. It is difficult to imagine anyone profiting by counterfeiting it. So amending the law to enable these super-low-cost drugs to be sold might reduce the counterfeiting that exists right now.

Another reason these less-regulated generics will do far more good than harm is that people who need them to live will be able to afford them. The media has reported on heart-wrenching stories of destitute people who are unable to pay for their prescription drugs. They either do without, or take a less-than-optimal dose. The availability of these free-market generics will enable virtually anyone to be able to afford their medications out of pocket.

EXAMPLE OF SUCCESSFUL REVOLT AGAINST FDA

A few years ago, news broke that the FDA had granted an exclusive monopoly to a company to sell a non-patented progesterone drug that prevents premature births.[65]

Healthy women naturally secrete huge amounts of progesterone during pregnancy, which helps maintain their uterine lining. To protect against premature births and miscarriages in women who don't secrete enough progesterone, doctors have for decades prescribed progesterone medications that were made by state-licensed compounding pharmacies. The cost per injection was around $20.

By granting orphan drug status to one company (KV Pharmaceutical), FDA rules banned all other forms of progesterone for this indication. The immediate impact was that the cost per injection of this progesterone drug was set to skyrocket to $1,500—or as much as $30,000 for a full-term pregnancy.[66]

An uprising over this price gouging forced the FDA to back down and state it "does not intend to take enforcement action against pharmacies that compound hydroxyprogesterone caproate."[67]

What the FDA is saying is that while it has the discretion to arrest compounding pharmacists for making this drug, it does not "intend to" do so.[68] After the FDA made this announcement, KV Pharmaceutical reduced the price to $690, which was still more than 34 times its previous free-market price. As of this writing, the cost of KV's progesterone drug is $779 per injection.[69]

It is unclear how private insurance and Medicaid will determine whether to pay $779 per injection for the version the FDA law says is the *only* one that can be legally sold, or continue paying for the much lower-cost compounded version.

Women who are denied access to this drug because of this regulatory quagmire face increased risks they will deliver pre-term babies. In these cases, the costs for intensive neonatal care can run into the hundreds of thousands of dollars per prematurely born baby, a price often borne by Medicaid or private insurance.

No country on earth can afford this kind of institutionalized corruption in which the chosen few pharmaceutical companies favored by the FDA reap extortionist profits as the nation collapses into a financial abyss.

This rare instance in which public backlash forced the FDA to back away from protecting a drug company's obscene profit reveals that citizens have the power to save this country from financial Armageddon.

FIGHT BACK AGAINST INSTITUTIONAL CORRUPTION

The United States of America faces a healthcare cost crisis that will render Medicare, Medicaid, and many private insurance plans insolvent. The shocking details about this country's inability to fund medical costs are no longer confined to my column in the *Life Extension Magazine®*. You are reading about them virtually every day in the mainstream media.

When terrorists attacked the United States in 2001, there were patriotic Americans who enlisted in the armed services. Many lost their limbs, their vision, and their lives.

No one has to engage in physical combat to save this country from the institutionalized inefficiencies and corruption that plague today's disease care system. All you have to do is enter STOPFDA.org into your computer's web browser. This will then automatically send a copy of these introductory chapters and a special letter to the President, your Representative, and two Senators.

It is that simple to take affirmative action to help save our country from the insolvency so many other countries chronically suffer with.

I sincerely hope that after reading this book, not one reader will fail to petition the federal government by logging on to www.STOPFDA.org.

We must unite and demand that Congress tear down the barriers of medical over-regulation that are destroying this nation's financial future.

MAGNITUDE OF IMPENDING HEALTHCARE COST CRISIS

In 2009, Medicare's unfunded liability was pegged at $37 trillion.[70] What that meant is that for the government to meet its future obligations, it should have had $37 trillion in a trust fund earning interest. But politicians constantly manipulate the numbers.

As this book was being written, there are four different "official" estimates of what Medicare's unfunded liabilities are, ranging from a low of $27.9 trillion to a high of $43.5 trillion.[71,72] Private government watchdog groups have pegged Medicare's true unfunded liability at over $100 trillion.[73,74]

The reason for these wild fluctuations is that in any given year, government officials can create "assumptions" out of thin air, like assuming doctors will take 21% pay cuts. Congress has not enacted these mandatory pay cuts, but bureaucrats sometimes pretend they have so that Medicare's true unfunded liability is understated.[75]

Despite these accounting gimmicks, a government report released in 2016 states that Medicare's hospital fund will go bankrupt in 2024, which is five years sooner than Medicare's trustees estimated the prior year.[76]

Be it $24 trillion or $100 trillion, the government does not have the money to pay its future Medicare obligations. Government also has no idea where the money will come from to cover unfunded liabilities for Medicaid, Veterans, and federal, state, and local employee sick-care plans it is on the hook for.

This book provides real-world solutions to spare the United States from healthcare cost-induced insolvency.

References

1. Available at: http://www.bloomberg.com/news/articles/2015-09-22/employer-health-insurance-costs-slow-as-workers-pay-bigger-share. Accessed November 7, 2016.
2. Available at: http://www.csmonitor.com/2003/1028/p01s02-usec.html. Accessed November 7, 2016.
3. Available at: http://www.gao.gov/products/GAO-16-357R. Accessed November 7, 2016.
4. Available at: http://www.taxpolicycenter.org/statistics/amount-revenue-source. Accessed November 8, 2016.
5. Available at: http://www.whitehouse.gov/the_press_office/remarks-by-the-president-to-a-joint-session-of-congress-on-health-care. Accessed November 8, 2016.
6. Available at: http://www.ncpa.org/pub/ba662. Accessed November 8, 2016.
7. The Long-Term Care Financing Crisis. Available at: http://www.heritage.org/research/reports/2013/02/the-long-term-care-financing-crisis. Accessed November 8, 2016.
8. Available at: http://www.economist.com/node/13983688?story_id=13983688. Accessed December 14, 2016.
9. Cancer Drug Avastin Linked to Death Risk. Available at: http://www.webmd.com/cancer/news/20110201/cancer-drug-avastin-linked-to-death-risk#1. Accessed November 8, 2016.
10. Rofecoxib (Vioxx) voluntarily withdrawn from market. Available at: http://www.cmaj.ca/content/171/9/1027.full. Accessed November 9, 2016.
11. Ranpura V, Hapani S, Wu S. Treatment-related mortality with bevacizumab in cancer patients: a meta-analysis. *JAMA*. 2011 Feb 2;305(5):487–94.

12. High-Priced Drugs: Estimates of Annual Per-Patient Expenditures for 150 Specialty Medications. Available at: https://www.ahip.org/wp-content/uploads/2016/04/HighPriceDrugsReport.pdf. Accessed December 12, 2016.

13. Oncologists: Cancer drugs have become too expensive: 11 of the 12 cancer drugs approved last year cost more than $100,000 per year. Available at: https://www.advisory.com/daily-briefing/2013/04/30/oncologists-cancer-drugs-have-become-too-expensive. Accessed December 12, 2016.

14. The Evils of Big Pharma Exposed. Available at: http://www.globalresearch.ca/the-evils-of-big-pharma-exposed/5425382. Accessed November 9, 2016.

15. Special-Interest Spending. Available at: https://www.down-sizinggovernment.org/special-interest-spending. Accessed November 9, 2016.

16. Available at: http://www.anh-usa.org/access-to-estriol-2/. Accessed November 9, 2016.

17. Slatore CG, Chien JW, Au DH, Satia JA, White E. Lung cancer and hormone replacement therapy: association in the vitamins and lifestyle study. *J Clin Oncol.* 2010 Mar 20;28(9):1540–6.

18. Maalouf NM, Sato AH, Welch BJ, et al. Postmenopausal hormone use and the risk of nephrolithiasis: results from the Women's Health Initiative hormone therapy trials. *Arch Intern Med.* 2010 Oct 11;170(18):1678–85.

19. Chen CL, Weiss NS, Newcomb P, Barlow W, White E. Hormone replacement therapy in relation to breast cancer. *JAMA.* 2002 Feb 13;287(6):734–41.

20. Beral V. Breast cancer and hormone-replacement therapy in the Million Women Study. *Lancet.* 2003 Aug 9;362(9382):419–27.

21. Cushman M, Kuller LH, Prentice R, et al. Estrogen plus progestin and risk of venous thrombosis. *JAMA.* 2004 Oct 6;292(13):1573–80.

22. Anderson GL, Judd HL, Kaunitz AM, et al. Effects of estrogen plus progestin on gynecologic cancers and associated

diagnostic procedures: the Women's Health Initiative randomized trial. *JAMA*. 2003 Oct 1;290(13):1739–48.

23. Manson JE, Hsia J, Johnson KC, et al. Estrogen plus progestin and the risk of coronary heart disease. *N Engl J Med*. 2003 Aug 7;349(6):523–34.

24. Shumaker SA, Legault C, Rapp SR, et al. Estrogen plus progestin and the incidence of dementia and mild cognitive impairment in postmenopausal women: the Women's Health Initiative Memory Study: a randomized controlled trial. *JAMA*. 2003 May 28;289(20):2651–62.

25. Vongpatanasin W, Tuncel M, Wang Z, Arbique D, Mehrad B, Jialal I. Differential effects of oral versus transdermal estrogen replacement therapy on C-reactive protein in postmenopausal women. *J Am Coll Cardiol*. 2003 Apr 16;41(8):1358–63.

26. Rossouw JE, Anderson GL, Prentice RL, et al. Risks and benefits of estrogen plus progestin in healthy postmenopausal women: principal results From the Women's Health Initiative randomized controlled trial. *JAMA*. 2002 Jul 17;288(3):321–33.

27. Weng JR, Tsai CH, Kulp SK, Chen CS. Indole-3-carbinol as a chemopreventive and anti-cancer agent. *Cancer Lett*. 2008 Apr 18;262(2):153–63.

28. Auborn KJ, Fan S, Rosen EM, et al. Indole-3-carbinol is a negative regulator of estrogen. *J Nutr*. 2003 Jul;133(7 Suppl):2470S–2475S.

29. Ashok BT, Chen YG, Liu X, et al. Multiple molecular targets of indole-3-carbinol, a chemopreventive anti-estrogen in breast cancer. *Eur J Cancer Prev*. 2002 Aug;11 Suppl 2S86–S93.

30. Yuan F, Chen DZ, Liu K, et al. Anti-estrogenic activities of indole-3-carbinol in cervical cells: implication for prevention of cervical cancer. *Anticancer Res*. 1999 May;19(3A):1673–80.

31. Bell MC, Crowley-Nowick P, Bradlow HL, et al. Placebo-controlled trial of indole-3-carbinol in the treatment of CIN. *Gynecol Oncol*. 2000 Aug;78(2):123–9.

32. Nakamura Y, Yogosawa S, Izutani Y, Watanabe H, Otsuji E, Sakai T. A combination of indol-3-carbinol and genistein synergistically induces apoptosis in human colon cancer HT-29 cells by inhibiting Akt phosphorylation and progression of autophagy. *Mol Cancer*. 2009 Nov 12; 8:100.

33. Fowke JH, Longcope C, Hebert JR. Brassica vegetable consumption shifts estrogen metabolism in healthy postmenopausal women. *Cancer Epidemiol Biomarkers Prev*. 2000 Aug;9(8):773–9.

34. Bioidentical Estriol Still under Threat. Available at: http://www.anh-usa.org/bioidentical-estriol-still-under-threat/. Accessed November 14, 2016.

35. Faloon W. FDA seeks to ban pyridoxamine. *Life Extension Magazine*®. 2009 Jul;15(7):7–12.

36. Voziyan PA, Khalifah RG, Thibaudeau C, et al. Modification of proteins in vitro by physiological levels of glucose: pyridoxamine inhibits conversion of Amadori intermediate to advanced glycation end-products through binding of redox metal ions. J Biol Chem. 2003 Nov 21;278(47):46616–24.

37. NephroGenex to "Pause" Pyridorin Development, Restructure, and Seek Strategic Alternatives. Available at: http://www.genengnews.com/gen-news-highlights/nephrogenex-to-pause-pyridorin-development-restructure-and-seek-strategic-alternatives/81252404. Accessed December 17, 2016.

38. The price of an EpiPen has skyrocketed more than 500% since 2009 — and senators are asking for answers. Available at: http://www.businessinsider.com/epipen-price-increases-about-500-percent-2016-8. Accessed November 14, 2016.

39. People are furious about the price of the EpiPen-here's how much it's increased in the last decade. Available at: http://

www.businessinsider.com/how-much-price-of-mylans-epipen-has-increased-2016-8. Accessed November 14, 2016.

40. It's Jaw-Dropping How Little It Costs to Make an EpiPen. Available at: http://time.com/money/4481786/how-much-epipen-costs-to-make/. Accessed November 15, 2016.

41. The $300 generic EpiPen from Mylan shows drug pricing is broken in the United States. Available at: https://mic.com/articles/152912/generic-epipen-mylan-half-price-300-dollars-still-shows-drug-pricing-crisis-in-the-united-states#. U1vUJo97O. Accessed November 15, 2016.

42. Drugmakers Turn Cheap Generics into Expensive Pills. Available at: http://www.wsj.com/articles/drugmakers-turn-cheap-generics-into-expensive-pills-1477849345.

43. The Latest in Atrocious Supreme Court Decisions—Only 2 Justices Stand Up for Your Rights... Available at: http://articles.mercola.com/sites/articles/archive/2011/03/22/betrayal-of-consumers-by-us-supreme-court-gives-total-liability-shield-to-big-pharma.aspx. Accessed November 15, 2016.

44. Why Drug Prices Are Out Of Control, Or Money Well Spent By Big Pharma. Available at: http://www.truth-out.org/opinion/item/21294-Why-Drug-Prices-Are-Out-Of-Control-Or-Money-Well-Spent-By-Big-Pharma. Accessed December 12, 2016.

45. "60 Minutes" Exposes the Horrific Moral Bankruptcy of Big Pharma's Cancer Drug Giants Like Novartis & Sanofi. Available at: http://www.feelguide.com/2014/10/06/60-minutes-exposes-the-horrific-moral-bankruptcy-of-big-pharmas-cancer-drug-giants-like-novartis-sanofi/. Accessed November 15, 2016.

46. 90% of Prescriptions Exposed As A Scam, Massive Corruption Uncovered Between Doctors & Big Pharma. Available at: http://www.feelguide.com/2014/01/12/90-of-prescriptions-exposed-as-a-scam-massive-corruption-uncovered-between-doctors-big-pharma/. Accessed December 12, 2016.

47. Online pharmacies step up efforts to reach your patients. Available at: http://www.acpinternist.org/archives/1999/11/epharm.htm. Accessed November 16, 2016.

48. The FDA versus the Life Extension Foundation. Available at: http://www.benbest.com/polecon/fdalef.html. Accessed November 16, 2016.

49. Zinman B, Harris SB, Neuman J, et al. Low-dose combination therapy with rosiglitazone and metformin to prevent type 2 diabetes mellitus (CANOE trial): a double-blind randomized controlled study. *Lancet.* 2010 Jul 10;376(9735):103–11.

50. Charles MA, Eschwege E. Prevention of type 2 diabetes: Role of metformin. *Drugs.* 1999 58 Suppl.1:71–3.

51. Libby G, Donnelly LA, Donnan PT, Alessi DR, Morris AD, Evans JM. New users of metformin are at low risk of incident cancer: a cohort study among people with type 2 diabetes. *Diabetes Care.* 2009 Sep;32(9):1620–5.

52. Rattan R, Giri S, Hartmann L, Shridhar V. Metformin attenuates ovarian cancer cell growth in an AMP-kinase dispensable manner. *J Cell Mol Med.* 2011 Jan;15(1):166–78.

53. Liu B, Fan Z, Edgerton SM, et al. Metformin induces unique biological and molecular responses in triple negative breast cancer cells. *Cell Cycle.* 2009 Jul 1;8(13):2031–40.

54. Anisimov VN, Egormin PA, Piskunova TS, et al. Metformin extends life span of HER-2/neu transgenic mice and in combination with melatonin inhibits growth of transplantable tumors in vivo. *Cell Cycle.* 2010 Jan 1;9(1):188–97.

55. Alimova IN, Liu B, Fan Z, et al. Metformin inhibits breast cancer cell growth, colony formation and induces cell cycle arrest in vitro. *Cell Cycle.* 2009 Mar 15;8(6):909–15.

56. Bodmer M, Meier C, Krahenbuhl S, Jick SS, Meier CR. Long-term metformin use is associated with decreased risk of breast cancer. *Diabetes Care.* 2010 Jun;33(6):1304–8.

57. Yurekli BS, Karaca B, Cetinkalp S, Uslu R. Is it the time for metformin to take place in adjuvant treatment of Her-2

positive breast cancer? Teaching new tricks to old dogs. *Med Hypotheses*. 2009 Oct;73(4):606–7.

58. Stanosz S. An attempt at conservative treatment in selected cases of type I endometrial carcinoma (stage I a/G1) in young women. *Eur J Gynaecol Oncol*. 2009 30(4):365–9.

59. Ben Sahra I, Laurent K, Giuliano S, et al. Targeting cancer cell metabolism: the combination of metformin and 2-deoxyglucose induces p53-dependent apoptosis in prostate cancer cells. *Cancer Res*. 2010 Mar 15;70(6):2465–75.

60. Wang LW, Li ZS, Zou DW, Jin ZD, Gao J, Xu GM. Metformin induces apoptosis of pancreatic cancer cells. *World J Gastroenterol*. 2008 Dec 21;14(47):7192–8.

61. Algire C, Amrein L, Zakikhani M, Panasci L, Pollak M. Metformin blocks the stimulative effect of a high-energy diet on colon carcinoma growth in vivo and is associated with reduced expression of fatty acid synthase. *Endocr Relat Cancer*. 2010 Jun;17(2):351–60.

62. Memmott RM, Mercado JR, Maier CR, Kawabata S, Fox SD, Dennis PA. Metformin prevents tobacco carcinogenin-duced lung tumorigenesis. *Cancer Prev Res (Phila Pa)*. 2010 Sep;3(9):1066–76.

63. Faloon W. Consumer rape. *Life Extension Magazine®*. 2002 Apr;8(4).

64. Growing problem of fake drugs hurting patients, companies. Available at: http://usatoday30.usatoday.com/money/industries/health/2010-09-12-asia-counterfeit-drugs_N.htm. Accessed November 17, 2016.

65. Available at: http://www.fda.gov/NewsEvents/Newsroom/PressAnnouncements/ucm242234.htm. Accessed November 17, 2016.

66. Available at: http://www.nbcnews.com/id/41994697/ns/health-pregnancy/t/premature-labor-drug-spikes/. Accessed November 17, 2016.

67. Available at: http://www.fda.gov/NewsEvents/Newsroom/ PressAnnouncements/ucm249025.htm. Accessed November 18, 2016.

68. Drug maker lowers price of Makena pregnancy drug to $690 per dose. Available at: http://articles.latimes.com/2011/ apr/01/news/la-pn-makena-price-cut-fda-20110401. Accessed November 21, 2016.

69. Available at: https://www.drugs.com/price-guide/makena. Accessed November 23, 2016.

70. The 81% Tax Increase. Available at: http://www.forbes. com/2009/05/14/taxes-social-security-opinions-colum-nists-medicare.html. Accessed November 22, 2016.

71. 2015 Medicare/Social Security Trustees' Report Analysis. Available at: http://www.finance.senate.gov/imo/media/ doc/2015%20Trustees%20Report%20SS%20Medicare.pdf.

72. The 2016 Trustees Report: Yet Another Warning to Congress and the President. Available at: http://www.heritage. org/research/reports/2016/07/the-2016-trustees-report-yet-another-warning-to-congress-and-the-president#_ftn14. Accessed December 13, 2016.

73. Treasury Data Reveals Federal Shortfall of $614,000 per U.S. Household. Available at: Available at: http://www. intellectualtakeout.org/blog/treasury-data-reveals-federal-shortfall-614000-us-household. Accessed November 22, 2016.

74. You Think The Deficit Is Bad? Federal Unfunded Liabilities Exceed $127 Trillion. Available at: http://www. forbes.com/sites/realspin/2014/01/17/you-think-the-deficit-is-bad-federal-unfunded-liabilities-exceed-127-trillion/#64c026bc10d3. Accessed December 13, 2016.

75. Senate passes SGR deal, averting 21% Medicare pay cut for doctors. Available at: https://www.advisory.com/daily-briefing/2015/04/15/sgr-reform-passes. Accessed December 13, 2016.

76. Congressional Research Service: Medicare: Insolvency Projections October 5, 2016. Available at: https://fas.org/sgp/crs/misc/RS20946.pdf. Accessed December 13, 2016.

Preamble

HOW PHARMACEUTICAL INTERESTS MANIPULATE CONGRESS INTO BANKRUPTING OUR HEALTHCARE SYSTEM

BEFORE READING THE REVEALING CHAPTERS in *Pharmocracy II*, it is critical to understand the magnitude of control the pharmaceutical industry wields in Washington DC.

The tragic result is the enactment of corrupt legislation that garners outlandish profits to those with political connections, while driving up healthcare costs to levels that are unaffordable by governmental and private entities.

The Medicare Prescription Drug, Improvement, and Modernization Act of 2003 is an egregious example of how Congress can be corrupted into passing laws that pour hundreds of billions of dollars in profits into Big Pharma, while hastening the financial collapse of our healthcare system.

For years, Life Extension® fought a brutal battle in an attempt to prevent what we abbreviate here as the Medicare Prescription Drug Act from passing in Congress.

This 1,000-page bill, written by pharmaceutical lobbyists, provided $395 billion of taxpayer subsidies over a ten-year period for the purchase of prescription drugs at full retail prices.[1–4]

Just imagine if you owned a business (like a pharmaceutical company) where you sold a product for $100 that cost you $5 to make. You are protected against competition by federal agencies that destroy those who make less expensive options (like alternative therapies) available. Your problem is that consumers cannot afford your overpriced product.

Most industries respond to these kinds of issues by initiating more efficient business practices and cutting prices. What if, instead of lowering prices, you influenced the federal government to use tax dollars to buy your overpriced product? That's exactly what the pharmaceutical industry accomplished when they enacted the Medicare Prescription Drug Act, with more pharmaceutical lobbyists in the halls of Congress that night than elected officials.[5]

Here is an excerpt from what was reported by CBS News's *60 Minutes* about this bill:

> If you have ever wondered why the costs of prescription drugs in the United States are the highest in the world or why it's illegal to import cheaper drugs from Canada or Mexico, you need look no further than the pharmaceutical lobby and its influence in Washington, DC. According to a new report by the Center for Public Integrity, congressmen are outnumbered two to one by lobbyists for an industry that spends roughly $100 million a year in campaign contributions and lobbying expenses to protect its profits.[6]

Since that time, federal lobbying exploded, hitting a peak of $273 million in 2009, while never dipping below $200 million in any year since then.[7]

OBSCENE PROFITS GUARANTEED TO BIG PHARMA

Enacted in 2003, the Medicare Prescription Drug Act prohibited Medicare from using its enormous purchasing power to negotiate lower prices.[8] That meant taxpayers were stuck with the tab of paying around 60% more than government agencies like the Veteran's Administration, which is "allowed" to negotiate drug price discounts.[9]

It is no coincidence that prescription drug prices skyrocketed after Congress enacted these tax dollar-funded laws. Pharmaceutical companies took full advantage by charging any price they wanted, and the federal government paid full retail price for eligible Medicare beneficiaries.[10]

A study on the effects of the Medicare Part D provision of the Medicare Prescription Drug Act cited the real-world benefits pharmaceutical companies received from lobbying for the bill's passage.

> Because of the passage of Medicare Part D, pharmaceutical companies generated millions of new customers who previously lacked prescription drug coverage. Moreover, the pharmaceutical industry defeated the reform measures they feared most: legalized importation of lower-cost medicines, governmental price controls, and easier market access for less expensive generic drugs.[11]

Evidently, Big Pharma's ultimate objective in lobbying for the passage of Medicare Part D was the engineering of legislation and regulation that both opens up the floodgates of federal spending on pharmaceuticals and limits competition in the drug market. An aim they have never stopped working toward, as is reflected in the legislation that followed the Medicare Prescription Drug Act.[12]

When the Affordable Care Act was negotiated, pharmaceutical companies agreed to lower Medicare prices somewhat and to kick in money to subsidize the program. In return, they were guaranteed millions of newly insured consumers whose health insurance companies were required by law to cover unlimited use of many expensive medications for the lifetime of the patient.[13]

Be it the Medicare Prescription Drug Act or Affordable Care Act, pharmaceutical companies reaped gargantuan profits as consumers got stuck paying higher insurance premiums, deductibles, co-pays, and taxes.

For certain procedures, health insurance policy holders are denied access to the doctor or hospital of their choice. In these cases, which we call "no-pays," even those with expensive health insurance are denied treatment their doctor says is medically necessary. In order to live, they must pay out-of-pocket. It's even worse for lower income individuals who cannot meet their annual deductible that often exceeds $4,000.

New "taxes" were enacted to pay for the premium subsidies the Affordable Care Act provided to middle and lower income Americans, along with an expansion of Medicaid for the indigent.

As should be apparent by what you've read so far, pharmaceutical interests benefit enormously while consumers are saddled with costs so high that living standards for most have been markedly reduced over this time period.[14]

HOW THE DRUG LOBBY WORKS

To fully grasp the influence that pharmaceutical lobbyists exert over the United States Congress, one only has to look at how the aforementioned Medicare Prescription Drug Act was enacted.

The insidious way this law came into being provides an intriguing window into how pharmaceutical influence causes Americans to overpay for prescription drugs and then plunders tax dollars to subsidize some of those who cannot afford the artificially inflated prices.

The Medicare Prescription Drug Act was passed at 3:00 a.m., long after most people in Washington had gone to sleep. Most members of Congress initially refused to vote for the bill, arguing it was too expensive and provided a windfall to the drug companies. The drug lobbyists went into overdrive, going as far as to threaten to support opposing candidates in future elections if certain members of Congress did not vote for the bill.[3,4,15]

Despite there being no surplus federal revenue available to fund the Medicare Prescription Drug Act, pharmaceutical lobbying prevailed over fiscal/ethical consciousness as Congress narrowly enacted this bill.

To add insult to injury, within two weeks of the bill's passage, Medicare released data showing the true projected cost of the bill would be $534 billion, instead of the $395 billion that Congress was misled into believing.[16]

In sworn testimony before Congress, it was revealed this $534 billion cost projection was intentionally withheld from Congress on orders from a Medicare official who went to work for a high-powered Washington, DC, lobbying firm ten days after the bill was signed into law.[6,17]

If these numbers don't appall you, just two years later, in 2005, the White House released revised budgetary figures showing the cost to the US Treasury of the Medicare Prescription Drug Act may have been as high as $1.2 trillion—three times greater than what Congress was misled to believe![18]

Outsiders who helped push through the Medicare Prescription Drug Act included many former members of

Congress who were registered lobbyists for the drug industry. Pharmaceutical companies have long been known to reward former members of Congress with lucrative employment contracts.[1,19-22]

In fact, Billy Tauzin, the congressman most responsible for pushing through the Medicare Prescription Drug Act, retired to a $2 million-a-year job as president of the Pharmaceutical Research and Manufacturers of America.[5] Fourteen other congressional staffers, congressmen, and federal officials also went to work for the pharmaceutical industry after the Medicare Prescription Drug Act was passed—a bill that poured one trillion tax dollars into drug company coffers.[5,13]

HIGH PRICE OF CITIZEN APATHY

The squalid facts behind passage of the Medicare Prescription Drug Act leave no doubt as to how much power the drug industry wields over us. While consumer groups like the Life Extension Foundation® tried to defeat this crooked legislation, the sad fact is that too many members of Congress betrayed their constituencies and capitulated to the drug lobbyists.

The Medicare Prescription Drug Act was enacted because the American citizenry remained oblivious to this conspiracy to pillage tax dollars that funneled hundreds of billions of additional profits to the pharmaceutical industry.

In a market free of government regulation, drug prices would collapse in response to competitive pressures. Instead, prescription drug prices remain excruciatingly high. When faced with the prospect of having to lower their prices, the pharmaceutical industry instead perpetrated schemes (like the Medicare Prescription Drug Act) that force virtually every American to subsidize their egregiously overpriced drugs.

If only a small fraction of the American public had voiced their outrage to Congress, the Medicare Prescription Drug Act would not have passed.

Now that we know the realities of what this and other shady Medicare/Medicaid programs are really going to cost, each taxpayer faces the prospect of paying thousands of additional Medicare tax dollars every single year. Yet even with higher taxes, Medicare's eventual date with insolvency is inevitable unless medicine is radically deregulated.

This book comprises only a fraction of articles I have written over the past 34 years to expose the charade of medical regulation that is slowly bankrupting our country.

Unlike other books of this nature, I propose real-world solutions that, if implemented, can save this nation from insolvency as it vainly attempts to offset the corrosive effects of healthcare regulations that breed institutionalized corruption.

As you read the chapters of this book, you will realize how Life Extension's early warnings have manifested into a harsh reality that can no longer be ignored.

References

1. A Political History of Medicare and Prescription Drug Coverage. Available at: https://www.ncbi.nlm.nih.gov/pmc/articles/PMC2690175/. Accessed November 10, 2016.
2. 2009 Annual Report of the Boards Of Trustees of the Federal Hospital Insurance and Federal Supplementary Medical Insurance Trust Funds, Table III.C19.—Operations of the Part D Account in the SMI Trust Fund (Cash Basis) during Calendar Years 2004–2018, Page 120 (Page 126 in pdf). Available at: http://www.cms.hhs.gov/ReportsTrustFunds/downloads/tr2009.pd. Accessed November 10, 2016.

3. The Congressional Budget Office (CBO) estimates that spending on Part D benefits will total $94 billion in 2017. Available at: http://kff.org/medicare/fact-sheet/the-medicare-prescription-drug-benefit-fact-sheet/. Accessed November 10, 2016.

4. Total expenditures of the program for 2008 $49.3 billion. Projected net expenditures from 2009 through 2018 are estimated to be $727.3 billion. Available at: https://www.ncbi.nlm.nih.gov/pmc/articles/PMC5095698/. Accessed November 10, 2016.

5. The Other Drug War II: Drug Companies Use an Army of 623 Lobbyists to Keep Profits Up. Available at: http://www.citizen.org/congress/article_redirect.cfm?ID=7827. Accessed November 10, 2016.

6. Steve Kroft Reports on Drug Lobbyists' Role in Passing Bill That Keeps Drug Prices High. Available at: http://www.cbsnews.com/stories/2007/03/29/60minutes/main2625305.shtml. Accessed November 10, 2016.

7. Center for Responsive Politics, Pharmaceutical/Health Products Industry Profile: Summary 2016. Available at: https://www.opensecrets.org/lobby/indusclient.php?id=H04&year=2016. Accessed December 22, 2016.

8. Medicare Prescription Drug, Improvement, And Modernization Act of 2003 Available at: http://www.gpo.gov/fdsys/pkg/PLAW-108publ173/pdf/PLAW-108publ173.pdf. Accessed November 11, 2016.

9. Hayes JM, Walczak H, Prochazka A. Comparison of drug regimen costs between the Medicare prescription discount program and other purchasing systems. *JAMA.* 2005 Jul 27;294(4):427–8.

10. Uncle Sam barred from bargaining Medicare drug prices, Senate candidate Tammy Baldwin says, blaming rival Tommy Thompson. Available at: http://www.politifact.com/

wisconsin/statements/2012/sep/04/tammy-baldwin/uncle-sam-barred-bargaining-medicare-drug-prices-s/. Accessed November 11, 2016.

11. Drotleff, Erich Andreas. "Medicare Part D Prescription Drug Benefit: Who Wins and Who Loses, The." Marq. Elder's Advisor 8 (2006): 127. Available at: http://scholarship.law.marquette.edu/cgi/viewcontent.cgi?article=1065&context=elders. Accessed December 22, 2016.

12. A Record Year for the Pharmaceutical Lobby in '07. Available at: http://www.heal-online.org/pharm062408.pdf. Accessed December 22, 2016.

13. Negotiating for Lower Drug Costs in Medicare Part D. Available at: http://www.ncpssm.org/EntitledtoKnow/entryid/2061/negotiating-for-lower-drug-costs-in-medicare-part-d. Accessed December 1, 2016.

14. Available at: Dilemma over deductibles: Costs crippling middle class. http://www.usatoday.com/story/news/nation/2015/01/01/middle-class-workers-struggle-to-pay-for-care-despite-insurance/19841235/. Accessed December 1, 2016.

15. Public Citizen report on how drug companies and HMOs led an army of nearly 1,000 lobbyists to promote misguided legislation and increase profits (June 22, 2004). Available at: http://www.citizen.org/congress/reform/rx_benefits/drug_benefit/. Accessed November 11, 2016.

16. Under the Influence: Drug Lobbyists' Role in 2003 Medicare Modernization Act. Available at: https://mlyon01.wordpress.com/2007/04/04/under-the-influence-drug-lobbyists-role-in-2003-medicare-modernization-act/. Accessed November 15, 2016.

17. The Lobbyist Who Made You Pay More at the Drugstore. Available at: http://billmoyers.com/story/the-man-who-made-you-pay-more-at-the-drugstore/. Accessed November 15, 2016.

18. Medicare Drug Benefit May Cost $1.2 Trillion. Available at: http://www.washingtonpost.com/wp-dyn/articles/A9328-2005Feb8.html. Accessed November 16, 2016.

19. Swarms of Drug Industry Lobbyists and Campaign Cash Stymie Bid to Restrain Medicare Prescription Costs. Available at: http://www.fairwarning.org/2016/10/swarms-drug-industry-lobbyists-campaign-cash-stymie-bid-restrain-medicare-prescription-costs/. Accessed November 17, 2016.

20. Available at: http://www.nytimes.com/2004/07/23/technology/23biotech.html. Accessed November 17, 2016.

21. Available at: http://www.nytimes.com/2004/12/16/politics/16drug.html. Accessed November 17, 2016.

22. Available at: http://query.nytimes.com/gst/fullpage.html?res=950DE3D71F3AF930A35751C1A9659C8B63&pagewanted=2. Accessed November 17, 2016.

The FDA:
Failure to Protect

The Food and Drug Administration is the oldest consumer protection agency in the United States. Established in 1906 with the passage of the Pure Food and Drugs Act, the agency has grown over time in its bureaucracy, its scope, and its authority. Today, the FDA is responsible for insuring the safety and effectiveness of a wide spectrum of products, including foods, pharmaceuticals, medical devices, cosmetics, electromagnetic emitting radiation devices, veterinary products, and more. This represents a huge percentage of the entire US economy. But does the FDA work in the consumers' best interest? Or is it working for the industries it is supposed to regulate? In the following articles, William Faloon exposes the shortfalls in the FDA and urges consumers to speak out for reform of this powerful agency.

FDA Suffers Major Legal Defeat In Federal Court

T HE **FDA** **STRICTLY REGULATES** what drug makers are permitted to say about their products. Until lately, what could be said was limited to what the FDA allowed. Recent federal court decisions involving the FDA have ruled against speech prohibition. The latest victory over FDA censorship occurred when a maker of prescription drug fish oil sued the FDA to make a health claim about fish oil's potential to reduce cardiovascular disease risk.[1] The FDA insisted it was illegal for the maker of this fish oil drug to state a coronary disease prevention claim until the FDA said so. Fish oil has long been known to lower blood triglyceride levels. The FDA does not dispute this. What the FDA questions is whether persistently elevated triglyceride levels increase heart attack risk.

This chapter explores the FDA's defeat in federal court and provides startling revelations as to why the FDA is not convinced of the vascular dangers posed by elevated blood triglycerides. What may surprise you is how backward thinking the agency responsible for regulating our health-care has become. What I've done here is weave the science behind heart disease and triglycerides together with the FDA's archaic interpretation of this data and the federal court's final decision. You're going to read how an independent party (a federal judge) saw through the FDA's charade and ruled against the agency based on scientific and Constitutional grounds.

Triglycerides are a type of fat that can be measured in blood. After eating, your body converts some calories it doesn't need to triglycerides that are stored in fat cells. Triglycerides are released from fat storage for energy production between meals. Your body also makes triglycerides. Triglycerides themselves are not a component of atherosclerotic plaque. High triglyceride levels, however, create metabolic disturbances that increase heart attack and ischemic stroke risk.[2]

The FDA acknowledges that triglyceride levels over 500 mg/dL are dangerous. The FDA allows a claim that fish oil drugs can reduce heart attack risk in people with triglycerides over 500 mg/dL. The scientific argument the FDA lost in federal court is whether persistently high triglyceride levels between 200 to 499 mg/dL are a vascular risk factor.

WHAT ARE OPTIMAL TRIGLYCERIDE READINGS?

Life Extension® has argued for the past 36 years that optimal triglyceride levels are below 100 mg/dL. The American Heart Association concurs with Life Extension's position on what ideal triglyceride levels should be.[3] To keep score, the box on the next page shows the upper-limit triglyceride numbers being debated by various groups:

Organization	Triglyceride Upper Limit
American Heart Association	Under 100 mg/dL
Life Extension®	Under 100 mg/dL
Conventional Refererence Value	Under 150 mg/dL
Food & Drug Admin. (FDA)	Under 500 mg/dL

As you can see, there is quite a difference of opinion on this issue. Fortunately, a federal judge ruled unconstitutional the FDA's position that a claim cannot be made for a health benefit when lowering triglyceride levels already below 500 mg/dL.

One of the judge's reasons for this favorable ruling is that the evidence supporting the triglyceride-lowering effect of fish oil is truthful and non-misleading,[4-6] as is the totality of scientific evidence that reduction in triglycerides can reduce vascular disease risk.[7-9] It helped that the FDA itself admitted these benefits of fish oil in the court proceedings. The agency nonetheless clung to its antiquated argument that it retained arbitrary power to censor the health claim, whether it is truthful or not! The judge disagreed that the FDA could prohibit truthful speech.

The FDA argued that they could deny this health claim for fish oil because " . . . recent scientific studies have left it unclear whether reducing the triglyceride levels of persons with persistently high triglycerides reduces cardiovascular risk." [10] The judge respectfully disagreed with the FDA's interpretation of the scientific literature.

WHY THE DEBATE OVER TRIGLYCERIDES?

In 1980, the *New England Journal of Medicine* published an article stating the evidence that triglycerides were an independent causative factor in vascular disease risk was "meager."[11]

We at Life Extension® vehemently disagreed, but our organization was so tiny back then that no one paid any attention. Despite several decades of research, there is still a controversy as to whether persistently elevated triglycerides by themselves (independently) increase heart attack/stroke risk.

It has been challenging to pinpoint the exact lethality of high triglycerides. One reason is that people with elevated triglycerides often present with low HDL, insulin resistance, obesity, and type II diabetes.[12–15] HDL beneficially removes cholesterol from arterial walls, while obesity and poor glycemic control are proven vascular risk factors.[16–20] So the question arises, if an obese and diabetic individual with low HDL suffers a heart attack and also has high triglycerides, was it the triglycerides or other factors that caused it? A quick answer in most cases is it was all of the above, plus other artery-clogging influences like chronic inflammation.

To further obscure the issue, high triglycerides are associated with dangerous small-dense LDL particles,[21] very low-density lipoproteins (VLDL),[22] and cholesterol-enriched remnant lipoprotein particles.[23] These are all known promoters of atherosclerosis.[24–26]

These and other confounding factors have made it challenging for the scientific community to agree on what triglyceride level predisposes people to cardiovascular diseases. Life Extension® takes a rather simplistic view of this. We have tested the blood of thousands of younger individuals. If they are normal weight, their triglyceride levels are often below 70 mg/dL. These young adults don't yet suffer outward vascular problems, and are full of vitality. So why would anyone view triglyceride readings of 200 to 499 mg/dL in older persons as acceptable? We at Life Extension® want blood profiles to resemble healthy young people, not older individuals who often suffer from systemic atherosclerosis.

FDA SAYS FISH OIL CLAIMS ARE "HARMFUL"

The maker of a fish oil drug called Vascepa® wanted to present scientific evidence to doctors that lowering persistently elevated triglycerides might reduce coronary artery disease risk. The FDA objected to this claim and argued that if doctors were told that lowering triglycerides below 500 mg/dL might reduce coronary risk, then this "would be potentially harmful to the public health, and [the] FDA would consider such conduct to be potentially misleading or potential evidence of intended use."[10]

The FDA defended its rationale that communicating this information about fish oil and coronary artery disease is potentially "harmful" because it " . . . could cause a physician to prescribe Vascepa® in lieu of promoting healthy dietary and lifestyle changes or prescribing statin therapy."[10] The FDA's position was that if a claim about the fish oil drug lowering coronary risks were allowed, then doctors might ignore other atherosclerotic factors and prescribe only fish oil. The FDA offered to compromise by stating that if the maker of the fish oil drug "agreed not to make the coronary heart disease claim, . . . there would no longer be a 'credible threat of prosecution,'"[10] as the fish oil would no longer be potentially "harmful," according to the FDA's logic.

HUMAN DATA REVEALS DANGERS OF HIGH TRIGLYCERIDES

Solid evidence about the dangers of triglycerides came from an analysis of a large and respected study (National Health and Nutrition Examination Survey, NHANES), that looked at all five components of metabolic syndrome, which include:

- Hypertension
- Insulin resistance

- Abdominal obesity
- Low HDL
- Elevated triglycerides

The results of the NHANES study showed that cardiovascular risk was most strongly associated with elevated triglycerides.[2] This finding, however, does not itself prove triglycerides are an independent vascular risk factor because other components of metabolic syndrome also inflict arterial damage. More persuasive evidence comes from a meta-analysis that found for each 88.5 mg/dL increase in triglycerides in men, there was a 32% higher risk of cardiovascular disease. After adjusting for HDL, there was still a 14% higher cardiovascular disease risk for each 88.5 mg/dL increase in triglycerides.[27]

In women, the dangers of higher triglycerides were more pronounced. For each 88.5 mg/dL increase in triglycerides, there was a 76% increased cardiovascular risk and 37% increased risk after adjusting for HDL.[27]

To put this data in perspective, the FDA says there is insufficient evidence to prove that triglyceride levels up to 499 mg/dL are dangerous. Based on findings uncovered by the first meta-analysis, waiting for triglycerides to reach the 499 mg/dL level poses an increased risk for cardiovascular disease of 63% in men and 167% in women.[27]

A second large meta-analysis (over 262,000 people) found a 72% increased risk of cardiovascular disease in those in the upper third triglyceride blood level compared to the lowest.[8] This study further discredits the FDA's argument that up to 499 mg/dL of triglycerides has not been proven hazardous, especially in light of Life Extension® and American Heart Association positions that optimal triglyceride levels are below 100 mg/

dL. Based on this large study, the 5-fold difference of opinion over what are safe upper-limit triglyceride levels means that those who choose to follow the FDA's recommendations may be at a 72% increased risk of today's leading cause of death.

Perhaps the strongest triglyceride data comes from a study involving 13,953 men aged 26 to 45 who were followed up for 10.5 years. Baseline triglyceride levels in the top quintile were associated with a 4-fold increased risk of cardiovascular disease compared with the lowest triglyceride quintile, even after adjustment for other risk factors, including HDL. An evaluation of the change in triglyceride levels over the first five years of this study and cardiovascular disease in the next five years found a direct correlation between increases in triglyceride levels and cardiovascular incidences.[28]

In world regions with lower cardiovascular risk (e.g., Spain, Japan, and Africa) triglyceride levels below 100mg/dL are commonly found.[29-31] Clinical trials consistently demonstrate the lowest risk of cardiovascular disease to be associated with the lowest fasting triglyceride levels.[28,32,33] To make matters worse, as Americans accumulate more body fat, average triglycerides have been steadily increasing. Overall, 31% of adult Americans have triglyceride levels over 150 mg/dL, a number that even standard reference labs say is too high.[3]

This data about the dangers of elevated triglycerides was argued for years in the federal court proceeding whereby the FDA threatened to bring criminal charges against the maker of a fish oil drug. The judge ruled against the FDA on scientific grounds, which I find rather bizarre. Why are federal judges put in the position of making medical decisions like this? Isn't that what physicians are trained to do?

FDA COMPARES FISH OIL TO "BLACKMAIL" AND "JURY TAMPERING"

The FDA contended it reserved the right to bring criminal charges against the maker of this fish oil drug based solely on truthful, non-misleading information the company sought to convey to doctors.

In an attempt to persuade the judge that communicating this off-label use was illegal and not protected by the First Amendment, the FDA analogized it to crimes such as "blackmail" and "jury tampering."[10] The judge did not accept the FDA's warped analogy.

The FDA made a number of other irrelevant arguments seeking to prevent this fish oil drug claim from being made, to which the federal judge remarked: "none is persuasive."[10]

HOW TRIGLYCERIDES ACCELERATE ATHEROSCLEROSIS

Triglycerides are a form of fat in the blood that are either used for cellular energy production or stored as body fat. Triglycerides are not part of human atherosclerotic lesions. What happens when triglycerides are persistently elevated is they can contribute to deadly low HDL and impede the ability of HDL to remove cholesterol from arterial walls.[12,34] Elevated triglycerides also promote the formation of byproducts that are highly atherogenic.[21-23,35] These triglyceride byproducts promote arterial inflammation and abnormal arterial blood clotting while impairing endothelial function and insulin sensitivity.[3,36-39] Triglycerides also have a deadly impact that contribute to foam cells accumulating in atherosclerosis lesions.[40]

This is why Life Extension® and the American Heart Association advise that triglyceride levels should ideally be below 100 mg/dL. It took a federal judge's order to prevent the FDA from bringing criminal charges against a company that wanted to promote its fish oil drug for use in people with tri-glyceride readings in the 200 to 499 mg/dL range.

WHAT CAUSES ELEVATED TRIGLYCERIDES?

Factors that elevate blood triglyceride levels include a sed-entary lifestyle, excess body weight (especially in the abdo-men), unhealthy dietary patterns, and low intake of marine-derived omega-3 fatty acids.[3,41] What the FDA fails to understand is the association between triglyceride elevation and the aging process. For example, only 9.5% of people aged 20 to 29 have triglyceride levels over 200 mg/dL, whereas the number jumps to 22.6% in persons 60 to 69 years.[3]

Higher triglycerides have been observed in type I and type II diabetics.[42-44] In type I diabetes, higher triglyceride levels correlate with poor glycemic control.[42] Elevated tri-glycerides predict progression toward type II diabetes in nondiabetics.[45]

In people of all ages, insufficient intake of omega-3 fatty acids contributes to higher triglyceride levels.[46] Fortu-nately, quality fish oil supplements are available with or without a prescription. Various genetic defects can lead to very high triglyceride levels,[47] and in these instances, everyone (including the FDA) agrees that fish oil supple-mentation is essential to protect against heart attack,[48-51] ischemic stroke,[51-53] and lesser-known problems caused by elevated triglycerides like pancreatitis.[54-56]

An absurd argument the FDA made in the federal court case was that if a fish oil drug were allowed to be promoted to people with triglyceride levels between 200 to 499 mg/dL, then healthy lifestyle/dietary changes would not be made, since patients would see their triglycerides drop in response to fish oil. The court rejected the FDA's argument that sought to circumvent the First Amendment. The federal judge ruled that the maker of this fish oil drug had a free speech right to convey factual information without having to fear FDA prosecution.

DIETARY FACTORS AFFECTING TRIGLYCERIDE BLOOD LEVELS

Huge numbers of clinical trials have been conducted to ascertain what components of the human diet elevate or reduce blood triglyceride levels. Data from these studies show how one's triglyceride level can be modestly lowered by reducing the type and amount of unhealthy dietary fats, cholesterol-rich foods, and trans fats. In a meta-analysis of 30 controlled feeding studies, a moderate-fat diet decreased triglycerides by 9.4 mg/mL, whereas type II diabetics consuming this same modest-fat diet showed a striking 24.8 mg/dL decrease in triglycerides.[57] This data indicates how dangerous it is for *diabetics* to excessively eat the wrong fats. Diabetics suffer multiple metabolic disturbances that preclude them from safely burning/storing dangerous fats that wind up in their bloodstream as triglycerides.

To help lower triglycerides while boosting beneficial HDL, all aging individuals should avoid added sugars and restrict total carbohydrate consumption to below 60% of one's diet. To demonstrate the danger of fast foods, a feeding study found that consuming a meal with 15 grams of fat boosted postprandial (after-meal) triglyceride levels by a modest 20%, whereas high-fat meals (50 grams of fat), including those served in popular fast-food restaurants, increased triglyceride levels by at least 50% beyond fasting levels.[58] While standard blood tests are usually done in the fasting state, a number of recent studies show that chronically high-after-meal blood levels of triglycerides and glucose are particularly dangerous.[59-61] This data adds to the growing body of evidence showing marked reductions in disease risk by following healthier eating patterns.[62–64]

Adherence to a Mediterranean-style diet lowers triglycerides 10% to 15% more than a strict low-fat diet.[65,66] Yet triglyceride reductions in response to dietary changes are not always as substantial as many aging people require. In response to reduced calorie intake, there are consistent reductions in body fat and blood triglyceride levels. The more body weight shed, the greater the decline in blood triglycerides. The percent reduction, however, does not always result in people achieving optimal triglyceride levels, which is why fish oil is so important.

MOST DIRECT WAY OF SLASHING TRIGLYCERIDES

Consumption of omega-3 fatty acids has shown the most robust and consistent reductions in blood triglyceride levels.[6,67] A comprehensive review of human studies showed that triglyceride levels dropped 25% to 30% in response to daily ingestion of 4,000 mg of marine-derived omega-3s.[5] This study found a dose-response relationship, with each 1,000 mg of EPA/DHA producing a 5% to 10% reduction in blood triglyceride readings. The effects of fish oil in lowering triglycerides are more pronounced for individuals with higher beginning triglyceride levels.

Studies on plant sources of omega-3s have not produced consistent triglyceride-lowering effects. That's because plant-derived omega-3 comes in the form of alpha linolenic acid that requires an enzyme (delta-5-desaturase) to convert alpha linolenic acid to EPA/DHA in the body.[68] Activity of the delta-5-desaturase enzyme diminishes with aging.[69] Plant-based chia, flaxseed, and walnuts are healthy to eat, but don't expect them to lower triglycerides the same as cold-water fish. When one ingests marine omega-3s, EPA and DHA are obtained directly without the need of enzymatic conversion. For the purpose of lowering triglycerides, omega-3s should come from marine-derived EPA and/or DHA, i.e. fish oil concentrates.

The American Heart Association recommends 2,000 to 4,000 mg EPA/DHA a day to lower triglycerides, providing that the capsules are taken under a physician's care. This recommendation is based on a large body of evidence showing triglyceride-lowering effects of marine-derived omega-3.[70–73] A person with blood triglyceride levels above 100 mg/dL can usually determine an appropriate omega-3 dose. Life Extension® recommends a Mediterranean-type diet and supplementation with about 2,400 mg of EPA/DHA for overall health, which includes maintaining triglyceride levels in optimal ranges. If triglycerides remain stubbornly high, then increase the amount of fish oil capsules and try to make healthier dietary and lifestyle choices.

FDA CONCERNED ABOUT ITS REGULATORY AUTHORITY

The FDA argued in the court case it lost that it had the authority to censor a claim that this fish oil drug might reduce coronary artery disease risk. The FDA warned that if the judge were to uphold the right of the fish oil drug maker to communicate this data to doctors, this would be a "frontal assault . . . on the framework for new drug approval that Congress created in 1962."[10] The FDA also argued it had not determined that the fish oil drug is safe and effective and therefore the FDA could bring criminal charges against the maker of this fish oil drug. The FDA said its enforcement against promotional statements for this fish oil drug would not prohibit speech and therefore not violate the First Amendment.

The maker of the fish oil drug countered that the FDA's threat to bring misbranding charges for off-label use was having a

"chilling" effect that prevented doctors from receiving consti-
tutionally protected speech. The fish oil drug maker asked the
judge to grant a preliminary injunction against the FDA from
taking enforcement action, or declaratory relief recognizing
their First Amendment rights.

The judge ruled in favor of the fish oil drug maker and
against the FDA on this Constitutional issue. He made it
clear that the court was not denying the FDA's power to regulate, but merely allowing for the maker of this fish oil drug
to communicate truthful and non-misleading speech under
the First Amendment.

THE PRESCRIPTION FISH OIL DRUG

The name of the drug the FDA lost its legal case on is Vas-
cepa®. Unlike fish oil, dietary supplements that contain
EPA and DHA, Vascepa® contains only EPA. The reason
for this is that while EPA and DHA both lower triglycerides, DHA omega-3 can slightly increase cholesterol. Since
cardiac patients often have cholesterol issues, a company
obtained approval from the FDA to market EPA-only fish
oil as an expensive prescription drug.

The FDA approved Vascepa® only in people with very
high triglycerides (over 500 mg/dL). When the company
promoted Vascepa® to doctors for use in patients with
triglyceride levels between 200 to 499 mg/dL, the FDA
threatened criminal charges because according to the
FDA, there was insufficient evidence that lowering persistently elevated triglycerides (200 to 499 mg/dL) would
produce a benefit to patients with coronary artery disease.
In response to exercising their First Amendment right
to inform doctors of the benefit in lowering persistently
elevated triglycerides, the FDA mystically transformed

Vascepa® (EPA-fish oil) into a misbranded drug that sub-jected the company and its employees to criminal charges. The company making Vascepa® filed a lawsuit against the FDA stating their claims were truthful and non-mislead-ing. According to the company, the FDA was chilling free speech by claiming the company's promotion of Vascepa® for use in people whose triglycerides were 200 to 499 mg/dL was illegal.

Recall that the American Heart Association and Life Exten-sion® believe that optimal triglyceride levels for protecting cardiovascular health are under 100 mg/dL. The FDA views are diametrically opposite to what is near consensus in the medical community, i.e. triglycerides levels should be no higher than 100 to 150 mg/dL of blood.

INSIDE THE FDA'S BRAIN

One of the FDA's scientific arguments against making a claim that fish oil reduces cardiovascular risks in peo-ple with persistently high triglycerides (200 to 499 mg/dL) is that clinical trials using other triglyceride-lowering thera-pies had no impact on this group of patients. An FDA advi-sory panel concluded

> that although. . . Vascepa® had reduced triglyceride levels in patients with persistently high triglycerides, there was "substantial uncertainty" whether reduc-ing triglyceride levels would significantly reduce the risk for cardiovascular events in such patients.[10]

We at Life Extension® do not see how these "other" triglyc-eride-lowering therapies relate to the vascular protective ben-efits conferred by fish oil. The FDA nonetheless argued this point as a reason for suppressing the First Amendment right of the maker of Vascepa®. The judge rejected the FDA's asser-tion. The FDA further argued this point stating:

These trials "failed to demonstrate any additional benefit" of such drugs, and although some later analyses had suggested that patients with high triglycerides may benefit from using such drugs, "this remains to be confirmed."[10]

The judge again rejected the FDA's argument. Here is what the FDA wrote as a threat to bring criminal charges against the maker of Vascepa® if it stated a benefit in lowering persistently elevated triglycerides:

This product [Vascepa®] may be considered to be misbranded under the [FDCA] if it is marketed with this change before approval of this supplemental application.[10]

In response to FDA threats of incarceration, the maker of Vascepa® brought a First Amendment lawsuit seeking to stop the FDA from prohibiting the company " ... from making completely truthful and non-misleading statements about its product to sophisticated healthcare professionals. ... ."[1]

In other words, the maker of Vascepa® did not seek to promote their fish oil to consumers, but only to doctors. The FDA contended dissemination of truthful, non-misleading information to doctors was nonetheless "illegal" without FDA "approval" of the claims. The FDA lost this argument and the federal judge issued a final order barring the FDA from bringing criminal charges against the maker of Vascepa®.

WHAT'S GOOD AND BAD ABOUT VASCEPA®

Vascepa® is marketed to doctors as a fish oil drug that lowers triglycerides without raising LDL cholesterol levels. To the physician, this may sound appealing compared to a competitive fish oil drug called Lovaza®, which contains EPA and DHA. If you chose to use an expensive fish oil drug, Lovaza® might be the better choice. That's because of peer-reviewed findings showing Lovaza® lowered triglycerides by a median of 51.6%, whereas Vascepa® lowered triglycerides by a median of 33.1%, compared to placebo in both cases. Therefore, the studies examined found Lovaza® to be about 56% more effective than Vascepa® at triglyceride lowering when comparing median percent changes.[74]

The one benefit that Vascepa® has as stated on their website is, "Vascepa®, EPA only, has been shown to lower triglycerides without raising LDL (bad) cholesterol."[75] What doctors may not take the time to comprehend is that there is far more to consider than simply LDL cholesterol levels when comparing Vascepa® (EPA only) with Lovaza® (EPA+DHA).

Five direct-comparison studies from a large meta-analysis found DHA was more effective in reducing triglycerides than EPA. The same analysis also found DHA led to a 4.49 mg/dL *increase* in HDL-C, while EPA did not.[76] Although LDL cholesterol may rise to some extent with EPA plus DHA supplementation, a shortcoming of relying on EPA alone is that DHA may reduce the atherogenicity of LDL. This is because DHA has been shown to significantly increase the size of LDL particles compared with EPA.[77] Larger, more buoyant LDL particles are less likely to clog arteries with deadly plaque.[78]

In a large trial comparing EPA (Vascepa®) plus statin therapy to statins alone, rates of sudden cardiac death and coronary death were not reduced by EPA.[79] In a separate large trial in which subjects were given EPA plus DHA (Lovaza®), a 45% reduction in risk of sudden death was observed, along with a 20% reduced risk of death from any cause.[80] However, not all trials of omega-3 fatty acids have shown these robust effects.[81,82]

International cardiovascular professional societies support the use of fish oil supplements.[3,83,84] The American Heart Association recommends 2 to 4 grams of marine EPA plus

DHA daily for high triglycerides.[3] What we at Life Extension® are most troubled by is the fact that patients taking Vascepa® are unlikely to take other fish oil supplements, and therefore suffer a deficiency of the DHA component of the omega-3 family. How important is DHA? To start with, it forms the major structural component of brain cell membranes. When looking at the overall health benefits of DHA compared to EPA, the clear winner is DHA. Some respected sources have even written that most people could derive virtually all of fish oil's benefits by taking only the DHA fraction.[76,85,86]

The cost for a one-month supply of Vascepa® is around $250. Lovaza® costs around $300 a month. The same amounts of omega-3s can be obtained from high-quality dietary supplements for a fraction of these prices. Even those with health insurance generous enough to cover prescription fish oil drugs will often find the co-pays for omega-3 prescription drugs exceed the low free-market price of high-quality fish oil supplements. Some insurance companies refuse to cover prescription drug fish oils and tell their policyholders to buy their fish oil from a dietary supplement company. With the federal government committing billions of dollars a year to cover the full retail prices of prescription drugs for lower income individuals, we suspect that this is where many of the sales for Lovaza® and Vascepa® will come from. As a taxpayer, you should be outraged.

THE FEDERAL JUDGE'S FINAL RULING

After years of costly litigation, thousands of pages of documents produced, and huge amounts of productive time squandered, the court ruled in favor of a qualified health claim that could be made for the fish oil drug (Vascepa®) without the company exposing itself to criminal liability for misbranding. The court based this ruling on the fact that the claim is truthful and non-misleading, that the FDA accepted this phrasing else-where in their regulatory labyrinth, and the First Amendment. So here is the claim that is now allowed to be made to doctors about this prescription drug fish oil:

> Supportive but not conclusive research shows that consumption of EPA and DHA omega-3 fatty acids may reduce the risk of coronary heart disease. Vas-cepa® should not be taken in place of a healthy diet and lifestyle or statin therapy.[10]

That's it. After years of protracted disagreement that led to full-blown litigation, the above statement is the primary out-come of this First Amendment victory over FDA censorship. In the ruling, the judge quoted from prior cases that "'secur-ing First Amendment rights is in the public interest'" and "'the government does not have an interest' in the unconstitutional enforcement of a law."[10] The judge's concluding remarks from this 68-page ruling are:

> Finally, there is no basis to fear that promoting Vas-cepa® for this off-label purpose would endanger the public health. Vascepa® is a fish oil product. And it is already widely prescribed to treat patients with per-sistently high triglycerides. The FDA has acknowl-edged that it has no evidence that Vascepa® is harm-ful—indeed, it volunteered that it would not object to Vascepa's being marketed as a dietary supple-ment. The balance of equities and the public inter-est both thus overwhelmingly favor granting relief.[10]

BECOME AN EMPOWERED PATIENT

Doctors are so inundated with new findings and suffo-cating bureaucracy that they cannot keep up with every aspect of medicine. A growing shortage of practicing phy-sicians mandates consumers take partial charge of their healthcare. When it comes to many of the known cardio-vascular risk factors, taking charge is not difficult. As it relates to triglycerides, you want your blood levels to be under 100 mg/dL. The comprehensive Male and Female Blood Test Panels offered by Life Extension® include a host of vascular disease markers, including triglycerides.

If your triglyceride result comes back over 100 mg/dL, you are welcome to bring this to the attention of your physician. You may also want to take some action on your own, such as increasing your intake of omega-3s and making lifestyle changes to safely push triglycerides (and other vascular risk markers) down. You can then proudly show your physician what you accomplished and spare his/her time for more important treatment issues you may face.

To order a comprehensive blood test panel, call 1-800-208-3444 (24 hours) or log on to LifeExtension.com/blood.

HOW A CONSUMER REVOLT PROTECTED SUPPLEMENTS AGAINST FDA CENSORSHIP

The FDA has long argued that the First Amendment to the United States Constitution does not restrict the agency from censoring truthful, non-misleading information.

The FDA contends their authority to limit free speech protects the public.

Back in the early 1990s, the American citizenry revolted against the FDA's attempt to ban dietary supplements. The result was passage of a federal law in 1994 that prohibited the FDA from censoring scientific information about nutrients shown to confer health benefits.[87]

This 1994 law did not extend to prescription drugs, even if the drug ingredient is identical to dietary supplements and available without a physician's prescription.

References

1. Available at: http://www.aboutlawsuits.com/wp-content/uploads/2015-5-8-Amarin-offlabel-lawsuit.pdf. Accessed February 9, 2016.

2. Ninomiya JK, L'Italien G, Criqui MH, et al. Association of the metabolic syndrome with history of myocardial infarction and stroke in the Third National Health and Nutrition Examination Survey. *Circulation.* 2004;109(1):42–6.

3. Miller M, Stone NJ, Ballantyne C, et al. Triglycerides and cardiovascular disease: a scientific statement from the American Heart Association. *Circulation.* 2011;123(20):2292–333.

4. Jacobson TA. Role of n-3 fatty acids in the treatment of hypertriglyceridemia and cardiovascular disease. *Am J Clin Nutr.* 2008;87(6):1981s-90s.

5. Harris WS. n-3 fatty acids and serum lipoproteins: human studies. *Am J Clin Nutr.* 1997;65(5 Suppl):1645s-54s.

6. Skulas-Ray AC, West SG, Davidson MH, et al. Omega-3 fatty acid concentrates in the treatment of moderate hypertriglyceridemia. *Expert Opin Pharmacother.* 2008;9(7):1237–48.

7. Kris-Etherton PM, Harris WS, Appel LJ, et al. Fish consumption, fish oil, omega-3 fatty acids, and cardiovascular disease. *Circulation.* 2002;106(21):2747–57.

8. Sarwar N, Danesh J, Eiriksdottir G, et al. Triglycerides and the risk of coronary heart disease: 10,158 incident cases among 262,525 participants in 29 Western prospective studies. *Circulation.* 2007;115(4):450–8.

9. Austin MA, Hokanson JE, Edwards KL. Hypertriglyceridemia as a cardiovascular risk factor. *Am J Cardiol.* 1998;81(4a):7b-12b.

10. Available at: http://www.fdalawblog.net/Amarin%20Decision%208-2015%20Off-Label.pdf. Accessed February 10, 2016.

11. Hulley SB, Rosenman RH, Bawol RD, et al. Epidemiology as a guide to clinical decisions. The association between triglyceride and coronary heart disease. *N Engl J Med.* 1980;302(25):1383–9.

12. Jeppesen J, Hein HO, Suadicani P, et al. Relation of high TG-low HDL cholesterol and LDL cholesterol to the incidence of ischemic heart disease. An 8-year follow-up in the Copenhagen Male Study. *Arterioscler Thromb Vasc Biol.* 1997;17(6):1114–20.

13. Ginsberg HN, Zhang YL, Hernandez-Ono A. Regulation of plasma triglycerides in insulin resistance and diabetes. *Arch Med Res.* 2005;36(3):232–40.

14. Carr MC, Brunzell JD. Abdominal obesity and dyslipidemia in the metabolic syndrome: importance of type 2 diabetes and familial combined hyperlipidemia in coronary artery disease risk. *J Clin Endocrinol Metab.* 2004;89(6):2601–7.

15. Kraegen EW, Cooney GJ, Ye J, et al. Triglycerides, fatty acids and insulin resistance—hyperinsulinemia. *Exp Clin Endocrinol Diabetes.* 2001;109(4):S516–26.

16. Bjornholt JV, Erikssen G, Aaser E, et al. Fasting blood glucose: an underestimated risk factor for cardiovascular death. Results from a 22-year follow-up of healthy nondiabetic men. *Diabetes Care.* 1999;22(1):45–9.

17. Whitmer RA, Gustafson DR, Barrett-Connor E, et al. Central obesity and increased risk of dementia more than three decades later. *Neurology.* 2008;71(14):1057–64.

18. Winter Y, Rohrmann S, Linseisen J, et al. Contribution of obesity and abdominal fat mass to risk of stroke and transient ischemic attacks. *Stroke.* 2008;39(12):3145–51.

19. Nicklas BJ, Cesari M, Penninx BW, et al. Abdominal obesity is an independent risk factor for chronic heart failure in older people. *J Am Geriatr Soc.* 2006;54(3):413–20.

20. Cucuianu M, Coca M, Hancu N. Reverse cholesterol transport and atherosclerosis. A mini review. *Rom J Intern Med.* 2007;45(1):17–27.

21. Austin MA, Breslow JL, Hennekens CH, et al. Low-density lipoprotein subclass patterns and risk of myocardial infarction. *Jama*. 1988;260(13):1917–21.

22. Berglund L, Brunzell JD, Goldberg AC, et al. Evaluation and treatment of hypertriglyceridemia: an endocrine society clinical practice guideline. *J Clin Endocrin Metab*. 2012;97(9):2969–89.

23. Nordestgaard BG, Benn M, Schnohr P, et al. Nonfasting triglycerides and risk of myocardial infarction, ischemic heart disease, and death in men and women. *JAMA*. 2007;298(3):299–308.

24. Hodis HN, Mack WJ, Dunn M, et al. Intermediate-density lipoproteins and progression of carotid arterial wall intima-media thickness. *Circulation*. 1997;95(8):2022–6.

25. Hodis HN, Mack WJ. Triglyceride-rich lipoproteins and progression of atherosclerosis. *Eur Heart J*. 1998;19 Suppl A:A40–4.

26. Austin MA, Krauss RM. LDl density and atherosclerosis. *JAMA*. 1995;273(2):115.

27. Hokanson JE, Austin MA. Plasma triglyceride level is a risk factor for cardiovascular disease independent of high-density lipoprotein cholesterol level: a meta-analysis of population-based prospective studies. *J Cardiovasc Risk*. 1996;3(2):213–9.

28. Tirosh A, Rudich A, Shochat T, et al. Changes in triglyceride levels and risk for coronary heart disease in young men. *Ann Intern Med*. 2007;147(6):377–85.

29. Plans P, Ruigomez J, Pardell H, et al. Lipid distribution in the adult population of Catalonia. *Rev Clin Esp*. 1993;193(1):35–42.

30. Nakanishi N, Okamota M, Makino K, et al. Distribution and cardiovascular risk correlates of serum triglycerides in young Japanese adults. *Ind Health*. 2002;40(1):28–35.

31. Bovet P, Romain S, Shamlaye C, et al. Divergent fifteen-year trends in traditional and cardiometabolic risk factors

of cardiovascular diseases in the Seychelles. *Cardiovasc Diabetol.* 2009;8:34.

32. Onat A, Sari I, Yazici M, et al. Plasma triglycerides, an independent predictor of cardiovascular disease in men: a prospective study based on a population with prevalent metabolic syndrome. *Int J Cardiol.* 2006;108(1):89–95.

33. Assmann G, Schulte H. Relation of high-density lipoprotein cholesterol and triglycerides to incidence of atherosclerotic coronary artery disease (the PROCAM experience). Prospective Cardiovascular Munster study. *Am J Cardiol.* 1992;70(7):733–7.

34. Third Report of the National Cholesterol Education Program (NCEP) Expert Panel on Detection, Evaluation, and Treatment of High Blood Cholesterol in Adults (Adult Treatment Panel III) Final Report. *Circulation.* 2002;106(25):3143.

35. Cohn JS, Tremblay M, Amiot M, et al. Plasma concentration of apolipoprotein E in intermediate-sized remnant-like lipoproteins in normolipidemic and hyperlipidemic subjects. *Arterioscler Thromb Vasc Biol.* 1996;16(1):149–59.

36. Ferreira AC, Peter AA, Mendez AJ, et al. Postprandial hypertriglyceridemia increases circulating levels of endothelial cell microparticles. *Circulation.* 2004;110(23):3599–603.

37. Liu L, Wen T, Zheng XY, et al. Remnant-like particles accelerate endothelial progenitor cells senescence and induce cellular dysfunction via an oxidative mechanism. *Atherosclerosis.* 2009;202(2):405–14.

38. de Man FH, Nieuwland R, van der Laarse A, et al. Activated platelets in patients with severe hypertriglyceridemia: effects of triglyceride-lowering therapy. *Atherosclerosis.* 2000;152(2):407–14.

39. Wang L, Gill R, Pedersen TL, et al. Triglyceride-rich lipoprotein lipolysis releases neutral and oxidized FFAs that induce endothelial cell inflammation. *J Lipid Res.* 2009;50(2):204–13.

40. Botham KM, Wheeler-Jones CP. Postprandial lipoproteins and the molecular regulation of vascular homeostasis. *Prog Lipid Res.* 2013;52(4):446–64.

41. Lungershausen YK, Abbey M, Nestel PJ, et al. Reduction of blood pressure and plasma triglycerides by omega-3 fatty acids in treated hypertensives. *J Hypertens.* 1994;12(9):1041–5.

42. Verges B. Lipid disorders in type 1 diabetes. *Diabetes Metab.* 2009;35(5):353–60.

43. Kreisberg RA. Diabetic dyslipidemia.*Am J Cardiol.* 1998;82(12a):67U-73U; discussion 85U-6U.

44. Krauss RM, Siri PW. Dyslipidemia in type 2 diabetes. *Med Clin North Am.* 2004;88(4):897–909, x.

45. Tirosh A, Shai I, Bitzur R, et al. Changes in triglyceride levels over time and risk of type 2 diabetes in young men. *Diabetes Care.* 2008;31(10):2032–7.

46. Harris WS, Connor WE, Inkeles SB, et al. Dietary omega-3 fatty acids prevent carbohydrate-induced hypertriglyceridemia. *Metabolism.* 1984;33(11):1016–9.

47. Pejic RN, Lee DT. Hypertriglyceridemia.*J Am Board Fam Med.* 2006;19(3):310–6.

48. Singh RB, Niaz MA, Sharma JP, et al. Randomized, double-blind, placebo-controlled trial of fish oil and mustard oil in patients with suspected acute myocardial infarction: the Indian experiment of infarct survival--4. *Cardiovasc Drugs Ther.* 1997;11(3):485–91.

49. Available at: http://www.fda.gov/SiteIndex/ucm108351. htm. Accessed February 15, 2016.

50. Bucher HC, Hengstler P, Schindler C, et al. N-3 polyunsaturated fatty acids in coronary heart disease: a meta-analysis of randomized controlled trials. *Am J Med.* 2002;112(4):298–304.

51. Zhang J, Sasaki S, Amano K, et al. Fish consumption and mortality from all causes, ischemic heart disease, and stroke: an ecological study. *Prev Med.* 1999;28(5):520–9.

52. Keli SO, Feskens EJ, Kromhout D. Fish consumption and risk of stroke. The Zutphen Study. *Stroke.* 1994;25(2):328–32.

53. Xun P, Qin B, Song Y, et al. Fish consumption and risk of stroke and its subtypes: accumulative evidence from a meta-analysis of prospective cohort studies. *Eur J Clin Nutr.* 2012;66(11):1199–207.

54. Park KS, Lim JW, Kim H. Inhibitory mechanism of omega-3 fatty acids in pancreatic inflammation and apoptosis. *Ann N Y Acad Sci.* 2009;1171:421–7.

55. Lei QC, Wang XY, Xia XF, et al. The role of omega-3 fatty acids in acute pancreatitis: a meta-analysis of randomized controlled trials. *Nutrients.* 2015;7(4):2261–73.

56. Foitzik T, Eibl G, Schneider P, et al. Omega-3 fatty acid supplementation increases anti-inflammatory cytokines and attenuates systemic disease sequelae in experimental pancreatitis. *JPEN J Parenter Enteral Nutr.* 2002;26(6):351–6.

57. Cao Y, Mauger DT, Pelkman CL, et al. Effects of moderate (MF) versus lower fat (LF) diets on lipids and lipoproteins: a meta-analysis of clinical trials in subjects with and without diabetes. *J Clin Lipidol.* 2009;3(1):19–32.

58. Dubois C, Beaumier G, Juhel C, et al. Effects of graded amounts (0–50 g) of dietary fat on postprandial lipemia and lipoproteins in normolipidemic adults. *Am J Clin Nutr.* 1998;67(1):31–8.

59. Bansal S, Buring JE, Rifai N, et al. Fasting compared with nonfasting triglycerides and risk of cardiovascular events in women. *JAMA.* 2007;298(3):309–16.

60. Batty GD, Kivimaki M, Davey Smith G, et al. Post-challenge blood glucose concentration and stroke mortality rates in non-diabetic men in London: 38-year follow-up of the original Whitehall prospective cohort study. *Diabetologia.* 2008;51(7):1123–6.

61. Glucose tolerance and cardiovascular mortality: comparison of fasting and 2-hour diagnostic criteria. *Arch Intern Med.* 2001;161(3):397–405.

62. Hu FB, Willett WC. Optimal diets for prevention of coronary heart disease. *JAMA*. 2002;288(20):2569–78.

63. Available at: http://www.heart.org/HEARTORG/HealthyLiving/HealthyEating/Nutrition/The-American-Heart-Associations-Diet-and-Lifestyle-Recommendations_UCM_305855_Article.jsp#.VsIPsBGFN9B. Accessed February 15, 2016.

64. Available at: http://www.ncbi.nlm.nih.gov/books/NBK11795/. Accessed February 15, 2016.

65. Rumawas ME, Meigs JB, Dwyer JT, et al. Mediterranean-style dietary pattern, reduced risk of metabolic syndrome traits, and incidence in the Framingham Offspring Cohort. *Am J Clin Nutr*. 2009;90(6):1608–14.

66. Vincent-Baudry S, Defoort C, Gerber M, et al. The Medi-RIVAGE study: reduction of cardiovascular disease risk factors after a 3-mo intervention with a Mediterranean-type diet or a low-fat diet. *Am J Clin Nutr*. 2005;82(5):964–71.

67. McKenney JM, Sica D. Role of prescription omega-3 fatty acids in the treatment of hypertriglyceridemia. *Pharmacotherapy*. 2007;27(5):715–28.

68. Welch AA, Shakya-Shrestha S, Lentjes MA, et al. Dietary intake and status of n–3 polyunsaturated fatty acids in a population of fish-eating and non-fish-eating meat-eaters, vegetarians, and vegans and the precursor-product ratio of α-linolenic acid to long-chain n–3 polyunsaturated fatty acids: results from the EPIC-Norfolk cohort. *Am J Clin Nutr*. 2010;92(5):1040–51.

69. Maniongui C, Blond JP, Ulmann L, et al. Age-related changes in delta 6 and delta 5 desaturase activities in rat liver microsomes. *Lipids*. 1993;28(4):291–7.

70. Covington MB. Omega-3 fatty acids. *Am Fam Physician*. 2004;70(1):133–40.

71. Calder PC. The role of marine omega-3 (n-3) fatty acids in inflammatory processes, atherosclerosis and plaque stability. *Mol Nutr Food Res*. 2012;56(7):1073–80.

72. Davidson MH. Mechanisms for the hypotriglyceride-
    mic effect of marine omega-3 fatty acids. *Am J Cardiol.*
    2006;98(4a):27i-33i.

73. Goodfellow J, Bellamy MF, Ramsey MW, et al. Dietary sup-
    plementation with marine omega-3 fatty acids improve
    systemic large artery endothelial function in subjects with
    hypercholesterolemia. *J Am Coll Cardiol.* 2000;35(2):265–70.

74. Bradberry JC, Hilleman DE. Overview of omega-3 fatty acid
    therapies. *Pharm Ther.* 2013;38(11):681–91.

75. Available at: http://www.vascepa.com/different.html#.
    Accessed February 15, 2016.

76. Wei MY, Jacobson TA. Effects of eicosapentaenoic acid versus
    docosahexaenoic acid on serum lipids: a systematic review
    and meta-analysis. *Curr Atheroscler Rep.* 2011;13(6):474–83.

77. Mori TA, Burke V, Puddey IB, et al. Purified eicosapentae-
    noic and docosahexaenoic acids have differential effects on
    serum lipids and lipoproteins, LDL particle size, glucose,
    and insulin in mildly hyperlipidemic men. *Am J Clin Nutr.*
    2000;71(5):1085–94.

78. Vakkilainen J, Steiner G, Ansquer JC, et al. Relationships
    between low-density lipoprotein particle size, plasma lipo-
    proteins, and progression of coronary artery disease: the
    Diabetes Atherosclerosis Intervention Study (DAIS). *Circu-
    lation.* 2003;107(13):1733–7.

79. Yokoyama M, Origasa H, Matsuzaki M, et al. Effects of
    eicosapentaenoic acid on major coronary events in hyper-
    cholesterolaemic patients (JELIS): a randomised open-label,
    blinded endpoint analysis. *Lancet.* 2007;369(9567):1090–8.

80. Verboom CN. Highly purified omega-3 polyunsaturated fatty
    acids are effective as adjunct therapy for secondary preven-
    tion of myocardial infarction. *Herz.* 2006;31 Suppl 3:49–59.

81. Johansen O, Brekke M, Seljeflot I, et al. N-3 fatty acids do not
    prevent restenosis after coronary angioplasty: results from

the CART study. Coronary Angioplasty Restenosis Trial. *J Am Coll Cardiol.* 1999;33(6):1619–26.

82. Nilsen DW, Albrektsen G, Landmark K, et al. Effects of a high-dose concentrate of n-3 fatty acids or corn oil introduced early after an acute myocardial infarction on serum triacylglycerol and HDL cholesterol. *Am J Clin Nutr.* 2001;74(1):50–6.

83. Howlett JG, McKelvie RS, Arnold JM, et al. Canadian Cardio-vascular Society Consensus Conference guidelines on heart failure, update 2009: diagnosis and management of right-sided heart failure, myocarditis, device therapy and recent important clinical trials. *Can J Cardiol.* 2009;25(2):85–105.

84. Available at: http://www.goedomega3.com/index.php/files/download/304. Accessed February 16, 2016.

85. Mori TA, Bao DQ, Burke V, et al. Docosahexaenoic acid but not eicosapentaenoic acid lowers ambulatory blood pressure and heart rate in humans. *Hypertension.* 1999;34(2):253–60.

86. Kelley DS, Siegel D, Vemuri M, et al. Docosahexaenoic acid supplementation improves fasting and postprandial lipid profiles in hypertriglyceridemic men. *Am J Clin Nutr.* 2007;86(2):324–33.

87. Available at: https://ods.od.nih.gov/About/DSHEA_Wording.aspx. Accessed February 9, 2016.

CoQ10 Wars

C ONGESTIVE HEART FAILURE contributes to about 310,000 deaths each year in the United States.[1] Over 5.8 million Americans suffer from this condition where the heart is unable to pump enough blood to meet the body's needs.[2] A study published late last year evaluated heart failure patients that supplemented with higher dose CoQ10 in addition to standard therapy. The results showed a 44% reduction in cardiovascular mortality in the CoQ10 group compared to the placebo arm receiving only standard therapy.[3] When this study looked at deaths from *any* cause, those receiving CoQ10 had a 42% reduction in all-cause mortality. Based on this study's findings, if all congestive heart failure patients properly supplemented with CoQ10, more than 120,000 American lives might be spared each year.

What's interesting about this study is that it showed that in order for CoQ10 to produce these robust lifesaving benefits, it had to be taken over an extensive period of time. Unlike cardiac drugs such as beta-blockers that produce an immediate effect,[4] CoQ10 must build up inside one's cells in order to induce clinical improvements. Health freedom activists may recall the jihad launched by the FDA in the 1980s–1990s that resulted in product seizures and criminal charges brought against those selling CoQ10.[5,6] As you're about to learn, the loss of life caused by the FDA's censorship is beyond astronomical. This chapter will describe how to properly use CoQ10 to achieve rapid benefits, and why it has taken so long for others to figure this out.

A lot of people think coenzyme Q10 was discovered in Japan because that is where it was first approved as a drug to treat heart failure.[7–9] The Japanese are one of the world's largest CoQ10 producers.[8,10] The reality is CoQ10 was first isolated from beef hearts at the University of Wisconsin in 1957.[9] This research was continued in collaboration with Professor Karl Folkers, who conducted research at Merck & Co., Inc., and later at Stanford Research Institute and the University of Texas at Austin.[11–14] Numerous positive findings on CoQ10 were published in the 1960s–1970s.[15–20]

It was not until 1983 when Americans first learned about CoQ10 in an article published by the Life Extension® Foundation.[21] The FDA's response was that CoQ10 could not be legally sold because it was a prescription drug that required the agency's approval. The FDA went as far as to say that CoQ10 posed an imminent health hazard. Life Extension's® CoQ10 was twice seized and twice returned after we mounted two successful legal actions to thwart the FDA's attempt to ban consumer access to CoQ10.

The perverse regulatory structure that the FDA operates under created two problems. It allowed an American invention (CoQ10) to be monetarily capitalized on by the Japanese at the expense of American consumers. Far worse, the bureaucratic impediments erected against CoQ10 caused millions of American deaths, which we'll document at the end of this chapter.

WHY CoQ10 CONFUSED CARDIOLOGISTS

Physicians in the US are used to drugs that provide an immediate effect. For instance, if a statin drug (such as Lipitor®) is prescribed, there is almost always a sharp drop in a patient's LDL cholesterol level. Antihypertensive drugs usually provide a quick blood pressure-lowering effect. Anticoagulant drugs (like warfarin) quickly thin a patient's blood. These kinds of fast-acting drugs are what doctors and the FDA are accustomed to evaluating. When CoQ10 came along, it seldom met mainstream medicine's expectation of a pronounced and immediate effect, especially in patients with congestive heart failure. So the knee-jerk reaction by the mainstream was that CoQ10 has no meaningful clinical benefit.

A recent study confirmed that it takes a considerable period of time for CoQ10 levels to build up to a point where significant clinical benefits occur, such as a 42% reduction in all-cause mortality. This study corroborates what was published decades ago in *Life Extension Magazine*. We at Life Extension® long ago discovered that low-dose CoQ10 administered to people with chronic disease did not provide needed benefit. It was clear that higher doses of more absorbable forms of CoQ10 were required.

FDA DENIED CoQ10 TO DR. LANGSJOEN'S PATIENTS

In 1992, the FDA and Texas Department of Health raided Austin Whole Foods and other retail outlets to seize their CoQ10.[30] This severely affected the ability of Dr. Langsjoen's heart disease patients to access coenzyme Q10. The basis for these raids was the FDA's contention that coenzyme Q10 was an unsafe food additive. Patients whose lives were being saved knew different.

The citizens revolted and protested the FDA seizures in every possible way. They alerted the news media, wrote hot letters to the FDA, congressmen, and senators, and phoned up the Texas Department of Health to protest. Sixty agitated patients and family members assembled at a local church to plan a strategy for keeping CoQ10 on the market. These CoQ10 seizures and the impact they were having on Dr. Langsjoen's patients was the subject of a detailed article, titled "Heartless Behavior," in the popular *Texas Monthly* magazine (June 1992 issue) which is still available online (http://www.texasmonthly.com/content/heartless-behavior).[30]

After a monumental struggle, the Texas Department of Health backed down and patients were once again able to obtain CoQ10 (in Texas). For heart failure patients whose lives hung in the balance, the ordeal was beyond stressful.

Those with cardiac issues that would like to become a patient of Dr. Langsjoen can contact his clinical practice at the following address and phone: Peter Langsjoen, MD, 1107 Doctors Drive, Tyler, Texas 75701; Phone: 903-595-3778.

PIONEERING WORK OF PETER LANGSJOEN, MD

Peter Langsjoen, MD, is considered one of the world's foremost experts in the use of CoQ10 to treat cardiac disease.[22] He conducts his research and clinical practice in Tyler, Texas, and is a long-standing member of our Scientific Advisory Board. What makes Peter Langsjoen unique among cardiologists is that he measures his patients' CoQ10 blood levels to ensure they are absorbing enough of the CoQ10 he prescribes to induce a clinical response. As reported seven years ago in *Life Extension Magazine*, Dr. Langsjoen observed that patients with advanced heart failure often fail to achieve adequate blood (plasma) CoQ10 levels, even when using high doses of conventional CoQ10.[23] Dr. Langsjoen found that in response to the administration of 900 mg of conventional (ubiquinone) CoQ10, advanced heart failure patients only increased their total CoQ10 blood levels to about half of what they should be.[23] In patients with congestive heart failure, much higher CoQ10 blood levels are needed to induce symptomatic and clinical improvements.

In healthy people, the ingestion of 900 mg of conventional ubiquinone CoQ10 is expected to raise total blood levels rather substantially. Dr. Langsjoen postulated on the reason ubiquinone fails to significantly increase CoQ10 blood levels in critically ill patients. He has seen his advanced patients suffer impaired absorption caused from intestinal edema, which precludes optimal absorption of ubiquinone CoQ10.[23]

Frustrated with the inability of even high doses of ubiquinone CoQ10 to meaningfully elevate blood levels, Dr. Langsjoen sought to evaluate the effects of a more absorbable form of CoQ10 called ubiquinol. Dr. Langsjoen evaluated advanced congestive heart failure patients that had been taking an average of 450 mg per day of ubiquinone and changed them to an average of 580 mg per day of ubiquinol.[23] The objective was to quickly elevate CoQ10 blood levels in these patients who were nearing cardiac death. Dr. Langsjoen's results showed that ubiquinol increased mean plasma CoQ10 levels from 1.6 ug/mL to 6.5 ug/mL—a 4.06-fold improvement over ubiquinone.[23] Previous published studies indicate that heart failure patients require higher CoQ10 blood levels to obtain significant clinical benefit.[24–26] In order to achieve these higher therapeutic levels, Dr. Langsjoen found ubiquinol CoQ10 was required.

What's regrettable is how few cardiologists paid attention to Dr. Langsjoen's remarkable findings that could have saved the lives of their heart failure patients. Dr. Langsjoen went on to comment that he sees his best results when ubiquinol is initiated *early* in the course of the disease, before severe damage to the heart muscle develops.

ROBUST IMPROVEMENTS IN CARDIAC FUNCTION

The ejection fraction test assesses the heart's pumping capacity by measuring how much blood is pumped after each beat compared with the amount of blood remaining in the heart.[23] Healthy people have an ejection fraction of 55–75%, while those with congestive heart failure often have values of 17–40%.[27-29] In a study conducted by Dr. Langsjoen, the mean ejection fraction improved from a dangerously low 22% up to 39% in ubiquinol-treated patients who had follow-up echocardiograms.[23] This represented a recovery of up to 77% in this critical measurement of cardiac output. The higher blood levels of CoQ10 and the improved ejection fractions were accompanied by remarkable clinical improvement in these advanced patients. Based on these findings, Dr. Langsjoen's scientific group concluded:[23]

> Ubiquinol has dramatically improved absorption in patients with severe heart failure and that the improvement in plasma CoQ10 levels is strongly correlated with both clinical improvement and improvement in measurement of left ventricular function.

An Update from Dr. Langsjoen

At a meeting of Life Extension's Scientific Advisory Board on April 25, 2012, Dr. Langsjoen confirmed his previous findings and advised healthy older people who were not supplementing with CoQ10 to take between 300–400 mg per day for the first month to fully saturate their cells, and then back down to a daily maintenance dose of 100–300 mg per day. Dr. Langsjoen stated at this meeting that younger people with healthy digestive tracks could probably benefit equally with ubiquinone or ubiquinol, but as one ages they should consider ubiquinol as it absorbs far better into the bloodstream.

For patients with congestive heart failure, Dr. Langsjoen recommends continuous high doses of ubiquinol to maintain the ejection fraction at values that correspond with overall improvement in cardiac function. In these heart failure patients, 200 mg of ubiquinol twice per day is a good dose, reliably achieving therapeutic plasma levels of CoQ10 higher than 3.5 μg/mL.

NEW STUDY CORROBORATES DR. LANGSJOEN'S RESEARCH

The study I discussed at the beginning of this chapter was published in the September 25, 2014, online edition of the *Journal of the American College of Cardiology: Heart Failure*. It described the effects of 300 mg per day of ubiquinone given to a large group of chronic heart failure patients. After 16 weeks of administration of this dose and form of CoQ10, there were no significant changes in measures of ejection fraction compared to placebo.[3] What the researchers discovered, however, is that when these chronic heart failure patients took 300 mg per day of ubiquinone for two years, there was (compared to placebo) a remarkable:

- 44% reduction in cardiovascular mortality.
- 42% reduction in all-cause mortality.
- 45% reduction in the number of hospital stays (some people consider hospitals worse than jail).
- 29% improvement in the proportion of patients seeing a beneficial change in their NYHA classification (a composite measure of heart failure severity).

These findings are earth shattering! They reveal that more than 120,000 American lives could be saved each year with the use of a widely available dietary supplement. The authors of this study concluded:

> Long-term CoQ10 treatment of patients with chronic heart failure is safe, improves symptoms, and reduces major adverse cardiovascular events.

These findings help corroborate Dr. Langsjoen's pioneering research where he used higher doses of a superior-absorbing ubiquinol CoQ10 to achieve quicker improvements in cardiac ejection fraction. Dr. Langsjoen sees improved heart function in as early as three months and almost always by six months of treatment with ubiquinol at 200 mg twice per day.

There are over five million Americans afflicted with congestive heart failure today. Many can't wait two years for a conventional CoQ10 supplement to improve their condition and slash their risk of dying. They need to initiate 400–600 mg of ubiquinol daily to increase their heart's ejection fraction as soon as possible.

There is now solid evidence from a large, randomized multicenter published trial showing remarkable benefits when 300 mg a day of CoQ10 is added to standard treatment over a two-year period. What makes this finding interesting is that many heart failure patients in the past tried a relatively small CoQ10 dose and if an improvement in ejection fraction did not happen quickly, they and their doctor would have felt CoQ10 to be ineffective. This helps explain why conventional cardiology has been slow to catch on to CoQ10's lifesaving benefits. To a patient suffering from chronic heart failure, this information is priceless!

NATIONAL CANCER INSTITUTE AND CoQ10

Most people associate CoQ10 as having beneficial effects for the heart, brain, and kidneys. Overlooked is data showing that CoQ10 has protective effects against several forms of cancer.

According to the National Cancer Institute's position paper:[31]

> Interest in coenzyme Q10 as a therapeutic agent in cancer began in 1961, when a deficiency was noted in the blood of both Swedish and American cancer patients, especially in the blood of patients with breast cancer.[32–34] A subsequent study showed a statistically significant relationship between the level of plasma coenzyme Q10 deficiency and breast cancer prognosis.[35] Low blood levels of this compound have been reported in patients with malignancies other than breast cancer, including myeloma, lymphoma, and cancers of the lung, prostate, pancreas, colon, kidney, and head and neck.[32,36,37]

The National Cancer Institute goes on further to state:

> Some of the accumulated data show that coenzyme Q10 stimulates animal immune systems, leading to higher antibody levels,[38] greater numbers and/or activities of macrophages and T cells (T lymphocytes),[38,39] and increased resistance to infection. [40–42] Coenzyme Q10 has also been reported to increase IgG (immunoglobulin G) antibody levels and to increase the CD4 to CD8 T-cell ratio in humans.[43–45] CD4 and CD8 are proteins found on the surface of T cells, with CD4 and CD8 identifying helper T cells and cytotoxic T cells, respectively; decreased CD4 to CD8 T-cell ratios have been reported for cancer patients.[46,47]

With a plethora of studies showing CoQ10's heart benefits, the data about its potential anticancer properties gets lost in the popular media.

BATTLES TO DEFEND AGAINST CoQ10 PROHIBITION

After we introduced CoQ10 in 1983, public demand for this nutrient soared. The FDA's response was to seek to ban it altogether because they deemed it to be a prescription drug that required government "approval" to be sold. Companies selling CoQ10 were raided and individuals (including us) were placed under intense criminal investigation at enormous cost to taxpayers. In 1987, FDA agents accompanied by armed US Marshalls (with guns drawn) kicked down our doors and proceeded to seize every bottle of CoQ10, every one of our newsletters, and any other nutrient (magnesium, fish oil, etc.) they deemed to be an "unapproved drug." We later filed suit against the FDA and won back all of the seized materials, though the supplements were spoiled and had to be discarded.

In 1990, the FDA conducted an armed raid against Highland Laboratories in Oregon and seized their CoQ10 and accompanying literature.[48] The owner of this company was criminally indicted and rather than face the expense and uncertainty of a trial, pled guilty and was placed on six months house arrest.[49]

Frustrated that we continued to offer CoQ10, the FDA went to a state pharmacy board and declared that nutrients like CoQ10 posed an imminent threat to the public's health and therefore had to be embargoed from sale to the public. At the FDA's behest, pharmacy board inspectors placed embargoes on our CoQ10 and that of another supplier of CoQ10 in the same state. We prepared a 300-page lawsuit against the pharmacy board attesting to the safety and efficacy of CoQ10. As a courtesy, we presented the lawsuit to the pharmacy board's attorneys and gave them the option of lifting the embargo before we filed the lawsuit. After reading the 300-page lawsuit that substantiated the safety and efficacy of CoQ10, the pharmacy board lifted the embargo against us (and the other company) and promised to never take the FDA's word at blind faith again. The state pharmacy board was clearly perturbed that the FDA deceived them about the safety of CoQ10.

We were later arrested at the behest of the FDA and fought a multiyear battle in which the US Attorney's Office eventually dismissed the charges that the FDA brought that sought to incarcerate us for life. To this day, the FDA tries to censor claims that CoQ10 can benefit heart failure patients, despite overwhelming documentation that this nutrient markedly reduces death rates when properly used.

HOW MANY AMERICANS HAVE NEEDLESSLY PERISHED?

Based on findings published in the *Journal of the American College of Cardiology* late last year, CoQ10 can reduce overall death rates in patients with congestive heart failure by 42%. The number of lives that could be saved if every congestive heart failure patient properly supplemented with CoQ10 is potentially over 120,000 each year. If you multiply the number of lives lost by the 30 years the FDA has been censoring information about CoQ10, the total comes to over 3.6 million dead Americans, which is more than all the American deaths suffered by all the wars this nation has ever fought. The chart on the next page documents the striking carnage caused by FDA censorship of CoQ10 compared to all military conflicts the United States fought, starting with the evolutionary War.

American Deaths Caused by CoQ10 Censorship Compared to Major Wars	
Premature Deaths Caused by CoQ10 Censorship (1984–2014) Based on findings published in the *Journal of the American College of Cardiology* (December 2014) showing all-cause mortality <u>reduction</u> of 42% in CoQ10 supplemented heart failure patients.	**3,600,000**
Total Military Deaths for Every War Fought (Itemized chart of every war below)	**1,426,640**
American Deaths from Every Major War	
Revolutionary War	25,000
War of 1812	15,000
Mexican-American War	13,283
Civil War	750,000
World War I	116,516
World War II	405,399
Korean War	36,516
Vietnam War	58,209
War on Terror	6,717

Based on these staggering statistics, it's hard to argue why the FDA retains authoritarian power over the American citizenry. With universal access to websites, those Americans who wanted to trust the FDA could easily log on to the FDA's website (www.fda.gov) to read the agency's position on a given nutrient, drug, or hormone. They could then compare what the FDA says with another government website (www.pubmed.gov) that provides easy access to published scientific papers. For example, if one enters into PubMed the terms "CoQ10 and congestive heart failure," 13 new studies appeared in 2016 and up to the time I finished this book in August, 2017. Yet the FDA continues to ignore this published scientific research by censoring health claims for coenzyme Q10.

A lot of Americans have tragically been killed in this country's many wars. Fear of terrorism has caused our government to spend trillions of dollars. Too bad our leaders don't realize that amending the Food, Drug and Cosmetic Act to strip the FDA of its dictatorial power would save many more American lives and reduce healthcare cost outlays. The numbers speak for themselves. If you ask which war caused the most American deaths, a person versed in history will name the Civil War. The harsh reality is that the CoQ10 Wars have resulted in far more American deaths. This catastrophic loss of life will continue until science is allowed to replace authoritarian edict in determining medical treatment protocols.

DON'T ABANDON CONVENTIONAL HEART FAILURE TREATMENT!

The dramatic mortality-reducing effect of CoQ10 should not tempt heart failure patients to abandon standard therapy that includes ACE inhibitors (such as enalapril), special beta blockers (such as carvedilol) and sometimes spironolactone (a mineralocorticoid-receptor antagonist).[50] In the hands of a competent cardiologist, there is now an arsenal of drugs that have caused a paradigm shift of improved survival in those stricken with chronic heart failure.

The *New England Journal of Medicine* (Sept 11, 2014) featured a review article of the massive improvements in survival that have occurred since 1986 when multidrug therapy is properly prescribed to heart failure patients.[51] What makes the CoQ10 study published in 2014 so impressive is that heart failure patients who were fortunate enough to be in the group that received CoQ10 with standard therapy reduced their risk of cardiovascular deaths by 44%. The standard therapy-only group, however, would have had markedly reduced cardiovascular mortality compared to no drug treatment. What this means in a nutshell is that conventional cardiac drugs significantly reduce the rate of dying from heart failure, but when CoQ10 is added, there is an additional 44% risk reduction.

We at Life Extension® do not hesitate to criticize the many FDA-approved drugs that are laden with harsh side effects and are only minimally effective. There are certain medications, however, with extensive track records of lifesaving efficacy that should not be avoided merely because of the many "bad actors" that litter the pharmaceutical marketplace.

References

1. Blank AE, O'Mahony S. (2007). *Choices in Palliative Care.* Springer Science+ Business Media, LLC.
2. Bui AL, Horwich TB, Fonarow GC. Epidemiology and risk profile of heart failure. *Nat Rev Cardiol.* 2011 Jan;8(1):30–41.
3. Mortensen SA, Rosenfeldt F, Kumar A, et al. Q-SYMBIO Study Investigators. The effect of coenzyme Q10 on morbidity and mortality in chronic heart failure: Results From Q-SYMBIO: A Randomized Double-Blind Trial. *JACC Heart Fail.* 2014 Dec;2(6):641–9.
4. Winkler C, Hobolth L, Krag A, Bendtsen F, Møller S. Effects of treatment with β-blocker and aldosterone antagonist on central and peripheral haemodynamics and oxygenation in cirrhosis. *Eur J Gastroenterol Hepatol.* 2011 Apr;23(4):334–42.
5. Available at: http://openjurist.org/978/f2d/560/dietary-supplemental-coalition-inc. Accessed October 17, 2014.
6. Available at: https://hiddenamerica.wordpress.com/category/fda/. Accessed October 17, 2014.

7. T Schrier. Kaneka Nutrients LP. Email interview. April 25, 2006.

8. Available at: http://www.sciencebasedmedicine.org/coenzyme-q10-for-heart-failure-the-hype-and-the-science/. Accessed October 17, 2014.

9. Tran MT, Mitchell TM, Kennedy DT, Giles JT. Role of coenzyme Q10 in chronic heart failure, angina, and hypertension. *Pharmacotherapy*. 2001 Jul;21(7):797–806.

10. Available at: http://www.nutraingredients-usa.com/Suppliers2/Leading-Japanese-CoQ10-supplier-to-exit-market. Last updated June 2, 2009. Accessed October 17, 2014.

11. Saini R. Coenzyme Q10: The essential nutrient. *JPharm Bio-allied Sci*. 2011 3(3):466–467.

12. Crane FL. The evolution of coenzyme Q. *BioFactors (Oxford, England)*. 2008 32(1–4):5–11.

13. Olson RE. Karl August Folkers (1906–1997). *J Nutr*. 2001 Sep;131(9):2227–30.

14. Available at: http://university-discoveries.com/university-of-texas-at-austin. Accessed October 17, 2014.

15. Yamamura Y, Folkers K, Yamamura Y (Eds) *Biomedical and Clinical Aspects of Coenzyme Q*. Elsevier, Amsterdam; 1977, pp.281–98.

16. Yamamura Y, G. Lenaz (Ed). *Coenzyme Q. Biochemistry, Bioenergetics and Clinical Applications of Ubiquinone*. John Wiley & Sons 1985; pp.479–505.

17. Choe JY, Combs AB, Saji S, Folkers K. Study of the combined and separate administration of doxorubicin and coenzyme Q10 on mouse cardiac enzymes. *Res Commun Chem Pathol Pharmacol*. 1979 June 24(3):595–8.

18. Okada K, Kitade F, Yamada S, Kawashima Y, Okajima K, Fujimoto M. [Liver cell injury of antineoplastic agents and influence of coenzyme Q10 on the cellular K+ and membrane PD in the rat (author's transl)]. *Nihon Shokakibyo Gakkai zasshi = Japanese J Gastro*. 1979 Apr 76(4):896–904.

19. Thiele OW, Hoffman K. Coenzyme Q10 in Brucella abortus Bang. *Die Naturwissenschaften.* 1968 55(2):86.

20. Thoroughgood CA, Combs GF, Farley TM, Redalieu E, Folkers K. Effect of folacin on biosynthesis of coenzyme Q10 from p-hydroxybenzoic acid in the chick. *Int Z Vitaminforsch.* 1968 38(5):466–72.

21. Available at: http://www.lef.org/magazine/2004/8/report_coq10/page-01. Accessed October 17, 2014.

22. Available at: http://www.bottomlinepublications.com/content/article/health-a-healing/exciting-new-health-benefits-of-coq10. Accessed October 17, 2014.

23. Langsjoen PH, Langsjoen AM. Supplemental ubiquinol in patients with advanced congestive heart failure. *BioFactors Oxf Engl.* 2008 32(1–4):119–28.

24. Langsjoen PH, Langsjoen AM. Overview of the use of CoQ10 in cardiovascular disease. *BioFactors (Oxford, England).* 1999 9(2–4):273–284.

25. Langsjoen PH. Potential role of concomitant coenzyme Q10 with statins for patients with hyperlipidemia. *Curr Topics Nutr Res.* 2005 3(3):149–58.

26. Langsjoen PH. Coenzyme Q10 in cardiovascular disease with emphasis on heart failure and myocardial ischaemia. *Asia Pacific Heart J.* 1998 7(3):160–168.

27. Available at: http://www.hrsonline.org/Patient-Resources/The-Normal-Heart/Ejection-Fraction#axzz3GPiCobPX. Accessed October 17, 2014.

28. Available at: http://my.clevelandclinic.org/services/heart/disorders/hfwhatis. Accessed October 17, 2014.

29. Watson RD, Gibbs CR, Lip GY. ABC of heart failure. Clinical features and complications. *BMJ.* 2000 Jan 22;320(7229):236–9.

30. Available at: http://www.texasmonthly.com/content/heartless-behavior. Accessed October 17, 2014.

31. Available at: http://www.cancer.gov/cancertopics/pdq/cam/ coenzymeQ10/HealthProfessional/page3. Accessed October 17, 2014.

32. Folkers K, Osterborg A, Nylander M, Morita M, Mellstedt H. Activities of vitamin Q10 in animal models and a serious deficiency in patients with cancer. *Biochem Biophys Res Commun.* 1997 May 19;234(2):296–9.

33. Lockwood K, Moesgaard S, Yamamoto T, Folkers K. Progress on therapy of breast cancer with vitamin Q10 and the regression of metastases. *Biochem Biophys Res Commun.* 1995 Jul 6;212(1):172–7.

34. Ren S, Lien EJ. Natural products and their derivatives as cancer chemopreventive agents. *Prog Drug Res.* 1997 48:147–71.

35. Jolliet P, Simon N, Barré J, et al. Plasma coenzyme Q10 concentrations in breast cancer: prognosis and therapeutic consequences. *Int J Clin Pharmacol Ther.* 1998 Sep;36(9):506–9.

36. Folkers K: The potential of coenzyme Q 10 (NSC-140865) in cancer treatment. *Cancer Chemother Rep.* 1974 24(4):19–22.

37. Folkers K. Relevance of the biosynthesis of coenzyme Q10 and of the four bases of DNA as a rationale for the molecular causes of cancer and a therapy. *Biochem Biophys Res Commun.* 1996 Jul 16;224(2):358–61.

38. Bliznakov E, Casey A, Premuzic E. Coenzymes Q: stimulants of the phagocytic activity in rats and immune response in mice. *Experientia.* 1970 26(9):953–4.

39. Kawase I, Niitani H, Saijo N, Sasaki H, Morita T. Enhancing effect of coenzyme, Q10 on immunorestoration with Mycobacterium bovis BCG in tumor-bearing mice. *Gan.* 1978 Aug;69(4):493–7.

40. Bliznakov EG. Effect of stimulation of the host defense system by coenzyme Q 10 on dibenzpyrene-induced tumors and infection with Friend leukemia virus in mice. *Proc Natl Acad Sci U S A.* 1973 Feb;70(2):390–4.

41. Bliznakov EG, Adler AD: Nonlinear response of the reticulo-endothelial system upon stimulation. *Pathol Microbiol (Basel)*. 1972 38(6):393–410.

42. Bliznakov EG: Coenzyme Q in experimental infections and neoplasia. *Biomedical and Clinical Aspects of Coenzyme Q.* Vol 1. Amsterdam, The Netherlands: Elsevier/North-Holland Biomedical Press, 1977:73–83.

43. Folkers K, Shizukuishi S, Takemura K, et al. Increase in levels of IgG in serum of patients treated with coenzyme Q10. *Res Commun Chem Pathol Pharmacol.* 1982 38(2): 335–8.

44. Folkers K, Hanioka T, Xia LJ, McRee JT Jr, Langsjoen P. Coenzyme Q10 increases T4/T8 ratios of lymphocytes in ordinary subjects and relevance to patients having the AIDS related complex. *Biochem Biophys Res Commun.* 1991 Apr 30;176(2):786–91.

45. Barbieri B, Lund B, Lundström B, Scaglione F. Coenzyme Q10 administration increases antibody titer in hepatitis B vaccinated volunteers—a single blind placebo-controlled and randomized clinical study. *Biofactors.* 1999 9(2–4):351–7.

46. Shaw M, Ray P, Rubenstein M, Guinan P. Lymphocyte subsets in urologic cancer patients. *Urol Res.* 1987 15(3):181–5.

47. Tsuyuguchi I, Shiratsuchi H, Fukuoka M. T-lymphocyte subsets in primary lung cancer. *Jpn J Clin Oncol.* 1987 Mar;17(1):13–7.

48. Available at: http://www.naturalnews.com/033280_fda_raids_timeline.html. Accessed October 17, 2014.

49. Available at: http://www.myopia.org/fdaraids.htm. Accessed October 17, 2014.

50. Available at: http://www.nytimes.com/health/guides/disease/heart-failure/medications.html. Accessed October 17, 2014.

51. Sacks CA, Jarcho JA, Curfman GD Paradigm shifts in heart-failure therapy—a timeline. *N Engl J Med.* 2014 Sep 11;371(11):989–91.

Horrific Conditions inside Drug Factories

'VE NEVER UNDERSTOOD why people traffic heroin or cocaine when higher profit margins are available manufacturing prescription drugs. In my early days I assumed that with their enormous price markups, at least minimum quality-control standards would exist at drug makers. How uninformed I was! As history has taught us, pharmaceutical companies don't care about their customer's health. It's not a part of their business model whether their drugs heal or harm. Their overriding concern is to make money.

Dietary supplement companies do not enjoy the gargantuan profit margins of regulated drug makers. Yet never have I seen such reckless disregard for consumer protection as has been exposed in the field of prescription drug manufacturing.

The FDA pretends to protect the public against contaminated drugs. The sordid facts reveal an agency incapable of acting in a rational manner, and when the FDA does something "after the fact," they often create worse problems. Such is the case of a company that made contaminated injectable drugs that sickened 745 Americans with 58 associated deaths at the time of this writing.[1] The FDA identified problems with this manufacturer as early as 2002, but dropped the ball into a state pharmacy board's lap that failed to act. FDA again identified dangerous problems in 2006, but once more failed to take actions other than send a "warning letter." The FDA now says it needs more power and money to do its job. What the FDA does not want the public to know is that the reason this shady manufacturer was able to take over such a significant part of the market is that FDA actions caused other companies to stop making certain injectable drugs.

The media was initially confused by this tragedy and blamed it on lack of regulatory authority. In this chapter, you'll see past this charade as you'll read how a drug factory pretended to be a compounding pharmacy. Particularly appalling is the FDA's inability to recognize that making as many as 17,000 vials of a drug all at once under filthy conditions was a far cry from custom-making one drug at a time per individual prescription in a sterile environment. The contamination problem, however, is not isolated to one bad drug maker. It turns out that these kinds of safety violations were routine at drug factories that the FDA had certified as being safe.

US DRUG FACTORIES IN "TERRIBLE SHAPE"

Here's how the *New York Times* described conditions inside FDA-registered drug factories:

> Weevils floating in vials of heparin. Morphine cartridges containing up to twice the labeled dose. Manufacturing plants with rusty tools, mold in

production areas and—in one memorable case—
a barrel of urine.[2]

The *New York Times* emphasized that these were not
reports about the injectable drug maker that was linked
to 745 cases of infection and 58 American deaths.[1] These
quality lapses were found at large drug companies whose
names are familiar to many Americans.[2]

When these problems were discovered, the FDA sent out
"warnings" to these companies. Instead of fixing the problems, many of these drug makers decided it was cheaper to
simply discontinue making the drug(s). The result was severe
shortages of the drugs cited by the FDA.[2] This opened up
the market for disreputable companies to make these same
drugs, who did so under the same kind of abysmal conditions the FDA found at large drug factories. The FDA would
like to take credit for stopping these problems, but in certain cases, it was people working at the drug factories that
came forward to complain about unsanitary manufacturing
conditions, or people dying from contaminated drugs, that
prompted FDA action. The sad fact is that some drug companies are so greedy they will not stop their highly profit-
able assembly lines to perform even the most rudimentary
sterilizing procedures.

CONTAMINATED INJECTABLE DRUGS

Fungal meningitis causes inflammation of the lining of
the brain and spinal cord that results in dreadful sickness
and sometimes death.[3] A drug factory made large quantities of a steroid (methylprednisone) that was injected into
the joints and spines of aging humans in chronic pain. It
provided temporary relief. The problem was this drug was
contaminated with a black fungus that infected those who
were injected with it.[4] Since injectable drugs bypass the

natural barriers afforded by an intact digestive/immune system, they have to be manufactured and maintained in a sterile environment to avoid killing patients. FDA inspections in 2002 and 2006 revealed injectable drugs being made under substandard (non-sterile) conditions at a drug factory. It was not until hundreds fell ill and scores died that the FDA took meaningful action.[5,6]

HOW THE FDA BUNGLED THE INVESTIGATION

The name of the company that made the fungus-laced injectable drug is New England Compounding Center (NECC).[4,5] It pretended to be a compounding pharmacy, but instead functioned as a drug factory. The FDA claims that it lacks adequate regulatory authority over compounding pharmacies, but FDA's inspection of NECC in the year 2002 revealed problems with sterility and other issues.[7] That same year, the FDA informed the Massachusetts State Board of Pharmacy of an adverse reaction to methylprednisone, which is the same drug that in 2012 caused the fungal-meningitis outbreak.[8]

Had the FDA done their job back in 2002, they would have forced NECC to register as a drug manufacturer and subjected NECC to stricter regulatory oversight, although that may still not have prevented the problems since FDA-registered drug makers were later found to have similar unsanitary facilities.[9] The FDA and Massachusetts state pharmacy board's most blatant failure, however, was to uncover horrific conditions inside NECC and take no practical steps to enforce safety compliance or shut down NECC before tragedy struck.[10]

GOOD MANUFACTURING PRACTICES OVERLOOKED

According to Massachusetts state regulators, the NECC drug factory failed to sterilize injectable drugs, something that is mandatory for a substance that is going to be injected into the body.[11] The regulators said that NECC didn't keep manufacturing equipment clean, operated a leaky boiler near the "clean room" where injectable drugs were packaged, and shipped products before receiving test results showing the products were sterile, which violates good manufacturing guidelines.[12,13] In addition, NECC did not test the manufacturing equipment used to sterilize injectable drugs on a timely basis according to regulators.[13] The result of these multitudes of quality lapses were injectable vials that contained black matter inside, which turned out to be the fungus that has been linked to 58 deaths so far.[1,10]

FDA INSPECTS AFTER CATASTROPHE

After hundreds had fallen ill from fungal meningitis, the FDA conducted a thorough inspection of NECC's drug factory.[14] The FDA's report cited greenish-yellowish discoloration on sterilization equipment and non-sterile raw ingredients. The FDA found that 25% of supposedly sterile vials were contaminated with greenish-black foreign matter and that 100% of these vials sent for analysis contained fungus.[14] The FDA noted that NECC was unable to provide documentation that its steam autoclave devices were capable of achieving product sterility, a critical factor when making injectable drugs.[10,13] In fact, FDA inspectors found greenish-yellow discoloration inside the one cleaning autoclave and a tarnished discoloration inside another.[13,15] NECC turned off its air conditioning in "clean rooms" from 8:00 pm to 5:30 am, which is improper because failing to keep clean rooms at low temperature and low humidity provides a fertile environment for fungal growth.[14,15]

Particularly troubling in the FDA report was documentation that NECC had found microbial contamination, but did not enact cleanliness procedures to neutralize this lethal threat.[14] Furthermore, "clean rooms" used to make injectable drugs had been identified by NECC's own staff as detecting bacteria and molds, but the FDA could find no evidence that the company acted to fix these lethal problems.[14] The FDA's belated inspection of NECC did nothing to prevent the suffering and death of hundreds of victims who contracted fungal infections from contaminated vials of methylprednisone injected into their spines and joints.[10]

FDA: FAILURE, DECEPTION AND ABUSE

My book titled *FDA: Failure, Deception and Abuse* was published in early 2010, but no one in Congress listened, and scores of Americans are dead because of the FDA's egregious ineptitude in the NECC fiasco.

CONGRESS CITES FDA FAILURE

The House and Senate held several hearings in November 2012 on the NECC tragedy. Congress wanted to know why the FDA didn't do more to prevent the production and sale of these tainted steroids. As anticipated, the FDA claimed that it didn't have enough authority to regulate pharmacies that compound drugs. FDA Commissioner (Margaret Hamburg, MD) warned that if Congress didn't strengthen legislation, another similar tragedy is inevitable. Dr. Hamburg stated before the House committee, [16-18] "If we fail to act, this type of incident will happen again. It is a matter of when, not if."

What Dr. Hamburg may not have expected was documentation that the FDA and the Massachusetts pharmacy board both repeatedly visited NECC and found problems, but the strongest action the FDA took was the issuance of a warning letter in 2006. In response to Dr. Hamburg claiming the FDA needed more "authority," one Representative responded, "We're just not buying it, doctor. . . . You lack the authority to do anything, yet you send a letter like this?" (In reference to FDA 2006 Warning Letter). This warning letter documented numerous violations of existing rules the FDA found in 2006, yet the FDA failed to take action until citizens started dying.

House members repeatedly berated regulators who failed to prevent the fungal meningitis outbreak, stating the FDA and Massachusetts state regulators both knew as far back as 2002 that there were problems at the pharmacy, which distributed more than 17,000 doses from contaminated lots of steroids. Dr. Hamburg was lambasted by House Committee members who stated:

> This is a complete and utter failure on the part of your agency.

> This is one of the worst public health disasters ever caused by a contaminated drug in this country.

> After a tragedy like this the first question we all ask is "Could this have been prevented?" After an examination of documents produced by the Massachusetts Board of Pharmacy and the US Food and Drug Administration, the answer here appears to be, "Yes."[18]

Other House members came to Dr. Hamburg's defense, arguing that a solution needed to be found instead of seeking to "prosecute the Food and Drug Administration."

SENATE HARSHLY CRITICIZES THE FDA

The day after the November 2012 House hearing, where the FDA asked for more authority, a bi-partisan staff of the Senate Health, Education, Labor, and Pensions Committee issued a report detailing how federal and state regulators knew nearly a decade before of serious safety concerns with the pharmacy (NECC) tied to hundreds of meningitis cases, but failed to act decisively. The report concluded that "bureaucratic inertia appears to be what allowed a bad actor to repeatedly risk public health."[19,20] While acknowledging the lack of clarity in what the FDA's role should be in regulating compounding pharmacies, the Senate cited plenty of evidence that the FDA should have taken action against NECC, which clearly was functioning as a drug factory. The Senate investigators wrote, "Both federal and state regulators were well aware that NECC and its owners posed a risk to the public health" and "repeatedly failed to demonstrate that the company could safely compound sterile products."[19] The Senate report uncovered an internal FDA memo in 2003 that concluded there was "potential for serious public health consequences if NECC's compounding practices, in particular those relating to specific sterile products, are not improved."[19] The Senate confirmed that methylprednisolone produced by NECC "had previously been a suspected cause of at least two cases with bacterial meningitis-like symptoms" in 2002, leading to an FDA inspection . . . with no meaningful action taken.[19]

Most Senators expressed skepticism the FDA could effectively use widened authority under any new law, one stating "the FDA has failed to use its existing authority . . ." with another stating, "This has been going on since 2002. . . . It took all this time, and nobody did anything."[20] Regrettably, some Senators still believe that giving the FDA more tax dollars will solve these issues of bureaucratic incompetence and mismanagement. At the Senate hearing, FDA Commissioner Margaret A. Hamburg conceded:

> Perhaps we should have been more aggressive,
> (referring to the FDA's failure to inspect NECC and

follow up on the 2006 warning letter). There was a lot of debate within the agency about whether to proceed.[20]

Senators repeatedly questioned the FDA's sending NECC a warning letter in 2006 and a letter in 2008 saying that it planned to inspect, but not following through until after the fungal meningitis outbreak occurred in late 2012.[19,21]

CBS NEWS ENABLES FDA TO TEMPORARILY DECEIVE PUBLIC

On March 10, 2013, CBS News' *60 Minutes* aired an emotional broadcast about the NECC tragedy that included interviewing victims who suffered horrific illnesses, along with family members of those who died.[22] *60 Minutes* accurately told this story about NECC-contaminated drugs that caused 58 deaths and over 700 serious illnesses.[1] What *60 Minutes* omitted was the fact that the FDA knew about this disaster-waiting-to-happen, but failed to stop it until Americans started dying in 2012. FDA officials were given free rein on *60 Minutes* to blame this catastrophe on a lack of regulatory authority. As you're learning here, the fault instead lies with bureaucratic ineptitude at the hands of the FDA and the state pharmacy board that permitted these lethal deviations in good manufacturing practices to occur.

Instead of blaming the FDA for ignoring this lethal problem, *CBS News* let FDA officials blame Congress for not giving the FDA more regulatory power. What the FDA does not want the public to know is that the reason this shady manufacturer was able to take over such a significant part of the market is that FDA actions caused other companies to stop making certain injectable drugs. *CBS News* overlooked the House and Senate investigations that documented FDA's egregious failings in the NECC matter.

FDA SAYS IT LACKS AUTHORITY . . .

But the FDA does have the authority. And it did in 2006, when the FDA inspected and sent a warning letter in effect telling NECC to stop manufacturing certain drugs or face legal action.[19]

In 2006, the warning came because NECC (pretending to be a compounding pharmacy) was found, among other things, to have failed to verify if supposedly sterile drugs met safety standards.[19]

Move forward to 2012 and NECC was not only still operating, but was selling tainted drugs manufactured under horrifically unsanitary conditions.[19] Where was the FDA? Why did they wait for Americans to die before doing their job?

CONGRESS STRIKES BACK AT THE FDA

On April 16, 2013, the FDA was subpoenaed to appear before Congress to account for why more wasn't done to protect the public against contaminated drugs made at NECC.[13,23] Congress wanted the FDA Commissioner to explain why she was not more forthcoming about the FDA failures during the House and Senate hearings held in November 2012.

According to the House Committee report on the NECC debacle:

- The investigation revealed what FDA Commissioner Margaret Hamburg did not disclose during the November 2012 hearing: FDA received a litany of complaints about NECC and its sister company, Ameridose, right up until the 2012 outbreak.[13]
- These complaints were related to the safety and potency of NECC and Ameridose products, issues that the FDA failed to routinely, if ever, inform the state about.[13]

- After reviewing more than 27,000 documents, we found a dramatically different picture than the one painted by the FDA during our initial hearing in November. We now know that doctors, patients, providers, and whistleblowers tried to warn FDA for years that NECC and Ameridose were operating as manufacturers and marketing their products nationwide without patient prescriptions.[13]
- The FDA was also warned about sterility and safety issues with the companies' products. Rather than do its job and protect the patients who were taking NECC and Ameridose drugs, FDA chose not to act.[13]

The box below contains highlights from the House Committee report showing that FDA failures contributed to the NECC disaster and how the FDA tried to cover up their own ineptitudes.

HIGHLIGHTS FROM HOUSE COMMITTEE REPORT ON FDA'S COVER-UP AND FAILINGS

On April 16, 2013, the House Committee on Energy and Oversight issued a report titled:[23]

FDA'S OVERSIGHT OF NECC AND AMERIDOSE: A HISTORY OF MISSED OPPORTUNITIES?

Here are some highlights from the Committee's report:

Since the (November 2012) hearing, the Committee has pressed FDA to produce all of its documents relating to NECC and Ameridose in order to obtain a full picture of FDA's inspectional history, oversight, and decision-making with respect to these firms. Only after being threatened with the possibility of a subpoena in a February 1, 2013, letter to Commissioner Hamburg, did FDA finally complete its production on March 21, 2013.

After reviewing these documents, Majority Committee staff believes there is a strong basis for Members
to pursue answers from FDA on whether this tragedy was preventable had the agency taken action
under its existing authorities to address the steady
stream of complaints it had received about NECC
and its sister company, Ameridose, since issuing a
Warning Letter to NECC in December 2006.

In 2017, Barry Cadden, owner and head pharmacist
of the New England Compounding Center (NECC),
was sentenced to nine years in prison for racketeering, racketeering conspiracy, mail fraud, and
introduction of misbranded drugs into interstate
commerce with the intent to defraud and mislead.

The FDA's inaction in the face of years of complaints and red flags associated with the safety of
drugs made by NECC had a tragic ending.*

*This entire document can be accessed at: www.lef.org/necc.

WHAT CONGRESS OVERLOOKED

What was not discussed in Congressional hearings was
the FDA's history of abusing and misusing whatever
authority Congress gave it. For example, when the FDA
first discovered problems at NECC (in 2002), it chose to
direct its resources to prosecuting a man named Jay Kimball, who sold a drug (liquid deprenyl) that harmed no
one. Jay Kimball remained in prison until 2015.[24] In 2006,
while the FDA did not think it needed to stop NECC's
lethal manufacturing practices, it somehow found the
time to censor claims by cherry growers that cited scientific studies on their website showing cherries conferred
health benefits.[25]

What few understand is how the FDA has historically abused its authority in a discriminatory manner. The new "authority" the FDA is seeking would enable the agency to pick out small, well-run pharmaceutical firms and regulate them out of business using minor technical arguments that have no bearing on safety.

GLAXO PAYS $750 MILLION FINE FOR QUALITY LAPSES

GlaxoSmithKline is the world's 4th largest drug maker, with annual sales of nearly $46 billion and profits of almost $9 billion.[26] In July 2002, the FDA sent a warning letter about quality problems uncovered at one of Glaxo's subsidiary manufacturers. The egregious problems, however, were not corrected despite additional FDA inspections that continued to turn up severe problems, including failure to safeguard against microbial contamination.[27] The FDA initiated a seizure action in 2005 to remove adulterated and improperly made drugs.[28] Horrendous problems persisted, however, until the Justice Department filed a criminal complaint against GlaxoSmithKline and stopped what could have been a human catastrophe.[29] In October 2010, GlaxoSmithKline agreed to plead guilty and pay a $750 million fine to resolve criminal and civil liability regarding the manufacturing deficiencies.[29]

GLAXO'S DEFECTIVE DRUGS

The defective drugs, manufactured between 2001 and 2005, were Kytril®, Bactroban®, Paxil CR®, and Avandamet®.[29] Kytril® is a sterile injectable anti-nausea medication used by cancer patients receiving chemotherapy or radiation. Bactroban is a topical anti-infection ointment used to treat skin infections. Paxil CR® is the controlled-release formulation of the popular anti-depressant drug Paxil®, and Avandamet®

is a combination of Avandia® and metformin. Avandia has since essentially disappeared from the market because of increased heart attack risks, though an FDA advisory panel recently recommended it be allowed to be prescribed to certain diabetic patients.[30] Years after FDA approval, Glaxo sent out a black box warning about increased suicide risks in users of Paxil®.[31] With the realization that cardiovascular disease is the leading cause of death among diabetics, and suicide a huge risk in depressed patients, the notion that the FDA approved drugs with these kinds of side effects borders on absurdity.[32,33] These lethal side effect issues, however, are irrelevant to the manufacturing lapses that occurred.

According to an employee who filed a lawsuit against Glaxo over these uncorrected defects, the water system was contaminated, the air system allowed for cross-contamination between products, the warehouse was so overcrowded that rented vans were used for storage, the plant could not ensure the sterility of intravenous drugs, and pills of differing strengths were sometimes mixed in the same bottles.[34] Although FDA inspectors had spotted some problems, most were missed.

Glaxo paid the $750 million fine and admitted that its subsidiary failed to ensure that Kytril® and Bactroban® finished products were free of contamination from microorganisms. It also admitted that its manufacturing process caused Paxil CR® two-layer tablets to split, which the company itself called a "critical defect," because potential distribution of tablets would not have any therapeutic effect and no controlled release mechanism.[35] Glaxo admitted that Avandamet® tablets did not always have the proper mix of active ingredients and, as a result, potentially contained too much or too little of the ingredient with the therapeutic effect.[29]

POTENTIAL LETHAL IMPACT OF GLAXO'S ABHORRENT LACK OF QUALITY CONTROL

One can only imagine the problems that would occur if a depressed individual took a powerful anti-diabetic drug like Avandia, which could inflict acute hypoglycemia. A former employee identified nine instances where the wrong pills were sold, including Avandia® mixed in packages of over-the-counter antacids like Tagamet®.[36] For chemotherapy patients who are immune-compromised, they could have easily succumbed to an infection without their oncologists ever suspecting it was linked to the anti-nausea drug Kytril, which was not tested to ensure it was free of microbial contamination.

NO JAIL TIME FOR GLAXO EXECUTIVES

Glaxo denies that any patients were ever harmed by the adulterated drugs they distributed in the United States and also denied that these kinds of problems occurred at its other drug factories. No one from Glaxo faced criminal charges. I again remind readers that Jay Kimball, who sold a clean product that harmed no one, was imprisoned for 13 years. One difference is that Jay Kimball had no money for an attorney and had to represent himself in court (or render himself insolvent defending against FDA's prejudicial accusations). Pharmaceutical behemoths like Glaxo, on the other hand, spend virtually unlimited money on lobbyists and lawyers and have not faced personal criminal liability for the misdeeds they allowed.

REPUTATION IN LIEU OF REGULATION

One reason why horrific quality issues occur at pharmaceutical companies is that few consumers know who makes their prescription drugs. When your doctor writes a prescription, you take it to your pharmacy and usually get a brown-colored bottle with pills inside. Seldom is the manufacturer's name stated on the bottle. Drug companies can thus run their manufacturing facilities with reckless abandon with little reputational risk. Dietary supplement companies, on the other hand, prominently state their name on the labels of their products. In a more sensibly regulated environment, better-operated pharmaceutical companies would prosper as their reputation for quality control became known. Unfortunately, today's Orwellian regulatory structure has created utter chaos, with retail pharmacies not knowing which generic manufacturer is going to make which generic drug at any given time.

As we investigated further into making generic drugs more affordable, we learned how dangerous the prescription drug marketplace has become, with counterfeiting, shortages, and quality problems more rampant than reported by the media. We would prefer that pharmaceutical companies place a higher value on their reputation and instill better quality standards. Instead, regulatory burdens are so cumbersome that quality control takes a back seat to pleasing bureaucrats who wield unbridled power, but lack the competency to recognize catastrophic problems as occurred with the contaminated steroids made by NECC.

HOW MUCH MORE FDA FAILURE WILL AMERICANS TOLERATE?

In 1906, a book called *The Jungle* was published that described appalling conditions inside America's meat packing industry. The revelations in this book resulted in the establishment of federal laws that mandated standards of strength, purity, and quality of foods and drugs. Conditions inside some of America's drug factories are eerily similar to those described in *The Jungle*, yet the FDA has been around for more than 100 years! How much longer is the public expected to wait before the FDA effectively spends its $4 billion annual budget on real consumer protection, as opposed to threatening walnut and cherry growers for claiming health benefits of their foods?

No matter how many times the FDA fails to protect consumers against contaminated drugs, there are no calls for meaningful reform. Instead of recognizing FDA ineptitude, cries ring out to give the FDA more money and power . . . as Americans perish from contaminated drugs the FDA had the authority to stop!

NO FREE MARKET!

What the public doesn't yet understand is that contaminated drugs are the result of draconian regulations that limit free-market competition. By restricting drug making to only those controlled by incompetent bureaucrats, the inevitable result will be shortages, poor quality, and high prices. As I write this chapter, one of the challenges in dealing with the NECC catastrophe is that there may be new shortages of injectable drugs because there are not enough drug factories in the US to meet patient demand. Shortages create opportunities for unsavory companies to dump even greater amounts of overpriced and contaminated drugs into the bodies of unsuspecting victims. This kind of problem would not continue in a free market, but ever-increasing regulations are exacerbating the problems of drug shortages, deadly manufacturing practices, and obscenely high prices.

References

1. Available at: http://www.cdc.gov/hai/outbreaks/meningitis-map-large.html. Accessed June 25, 2013.
2. Available at: https://www.nytimes.com/2012/10/18/business/drug-makers-stalled-in-a-cycle-of-quality-lapses-and-shortages.html?pagewanted=all. Accessed June 13, 2013.
3. Available at: http://www.cdc.gov/meningitis/fungal.html. Accessed June 20, 2013.
4. Available at: http://www.nejm.org/doi/full/10.1056/NEJMra1212617?query=featured_meningitis. Accessed June 13, 2013.
5. Available at: http://www.upi.com/Health_News/2012/11/13/Meningitis-pharmacy-had-many-violations/UPI-28381352863651/. Accessed June 13, 2013.
6. Available at: http://www.washingtonpost.com/national/health-science/previous-fungal-meningitis-outbreak-a-decade-ago-resulted-in-no-oversight-changes/2012/11/05/8417d84e-1fa8-11e2-9cd5-b55c38388962_story.html. Accessed June 13, 2013.
7. Available at: http://finance.yahoo.com/news/fda-seeks-more-authority-amid-meningitis-outbreak-225136817--finance.html. Accessed June 13, 2013.
8. Available at: http://www.reuters.com/article/2012/10/23/us-usa-health-meningitis-congress-idUSBRE89M00820121023. Accessed June 20, 2013.
9. Available at: http://www.nytimes.com/2012/10/18/business/drug-makers-stalled-in-a-cycle-of-quality-lapses-and-shortages.html?pagewanted=all. Accessed June 13, 2013.
10. Available at: http://online.wsj.com/article/SB10001424052970203406404578075092760806164.html. Accessed June 13, 2013.
11. Available at: http://www.mass.gov/eohhs/docs/dph/quality/boards/necc/necc-preliminary-report-10-23-2012.pdf. Accessed June 27, 2013.

12. Available at: http://foodpoisoningbulletin.com/2012/necc-methylprednisolone-acetate-linked-to-meningitis-outbreak-evidence-drug-made-under-insanitary-conditions/. Accessed June 20, 2013.
13. Available at: http://energycommerce.house.gov/press-release/committee-report-meningitis-outbreak-chronicles-fdas-missed-opportunities-to-protect-public-health. Accessed June 21, 2013.
14. Available at: http://www.fda.gov/downloads/AboutFDA/CentersOffices/OfficeofGlobalRegulatoryOperationsandPolicy/ORA/ORAElectronicReadingRoom/UCM325980.pdf. Accessed June 13, 2013.
15. Available at: http://www.nytimes.com/2012/10/27/health/fda-finds-unsanitary-conditions-at-new-england-compounding-center.html?pagewanted=all. Accessed June 14, 2013.
16. Available at: http://www.reuters.com/article/2012/11/14/us-usa-health-meningitis-widow-idUSBRE8AD13020121114. Accessed June 14, 2013.
17. Available at: http://www.nytimes.com/2012/11/15/health/fda-asking-for-more-control-over-drug-compounding.html?_r=0. Accessed June 14, 2013.
18. Available at: http://www.nbcnews.com/health/pharmacy-owner-refuses-testify-about-fungal-outbreak-1C7055774?franchiseSlug=healthmain. Accessed June 14, 2013.
19. Available at: http://www.help.senate.gov/imo/media/doc/11_15_ 12%20HELP%20Staff%20Report%20on%20Meningitis%20Outbreak.pdf. Accessed June 14, 2013.
20. Available at: http://stream.wsj.com/story/latest-headlines/SS-2-63399/SS-2-102550/. Accessed June 14, 2013.
21. Available at: http://www.fda.gov/ICECI/EnforcementActions/WarningLetters/2006/ucm076196.htm. Accessed June 14, 2013.

22. Available at: http://www.cbsnews.com/8301-18560_162-57573175/meningitis-whistleblower-on-60-minutes/. Accessed June 14, 2013.

23. Available at: http://energycommerce.house.gov/sites/republicans.energycommerce.house.gov/files/analysis/20130416Meningitis.pdf. Accessed June 17, 2013.

24. Available at: http://www.lef.org/magazine/mag2004/aug2004_report_prisons_03.htm?source=search&key= Jay%20Kimball. Accessed June 17, 2013.

25. Available at: http://usatoday30.usatoday.com/news/health/2006-03-19-cherry-warnings_x.htm?csp=34. Accessed June 17, 2013.

26. Available at: http://www.forbes.com/lists/2010/18/global-2000-10_The-Global-2000_Sales_2.html. Accessed June 21, 2013.

27. Available at: http://www.fda.gov/downloads/iceci/enforcementactions/enforcementstory/enforcementstoryarchive/ucm091066.pdf. Accessed June 17, 2013.

28. Available at: http://www.fda.gov/NewsEvents/Newsroom/PressAnnouncements/2005/ucm108418.htm. Accessed June 17, 2013.

29. Available at: http://www.justice.gov/opa/pr/2010/October/10-civ-1205.html. Accessed June 17, 2013.

30. Available at: http://www.findavandiahelp.com/avandia_fda. Accessed June 17, 2013.

31. Available at: http://www.justice.gov/opa/pr/2012/July/12-civ-842.html. Accessed June 18, 2013.

32. Available at: http://www.world-heart-federation.org/cardiovascular-health/cardiovascular-disease-risk-factors/diabetes/. Accessed June 15, 2013.

33. Available at: http://www.webmd.com/depression/guide/depression-recognizing-signs-of-suicide. Accessed June 18, 2013.

34. Available at: http://www.nytimes.com/2010/10/27/business/27drug.html?pagewanted=all. Accessed June 18, 2013.

35. Available at: http://chiefofficers.net/888333888/cms/index.php/news/industries/health_care _pharma/pharmaceuticals/health_gsk_pays_usd750_million_fine_and_penalties_in_usa. Accessed June 15, 2013.

36. Available at: http://www.cbsnews.com/8301-18560_162-7195247.html. Accessed June 18, 2013.

Metformin Makes Headline News

ETFORMIN IS THE FIRST-LINE DRUG OF CHOICE in the treatment of type II diabetes. It was first approved in Europe in 1958.[1] Americans had to wait until 1995 to legally obtain metformin.[1] The holdup in approving metformin goes beyond the FDA. It is an indictment of a political/legal system that will forever cause needless suffering and death unless substantively changed.

When Life Extension® informed Americans about drugs like metformin in the 1980s, the FDA did everything in its power to incarcerate me and shut down our Foundation.[2] FDA propaganda at the time was that consumers needed to be "protected" against "unproven" therapies. As history has since proven, the result of the FDA's embargo has been unparalleled human carnage. So called "consumer protection" translated into ailing Americans being denied access to therapies that the FDA now claims are essential to saving lives.

Today's major problem is not drugs available in other countries that Americans can't access. Instead, it is a political/legal system that suffocates medical innovation. Headline news stories earlier this year touted the anti-cancer effects of metformin, data that Foundation members were alerted to long ago.[3] The problem is that it is illegal for metformin manufacturers to promote this drug to cancer patients or oncologists. It's also illegal to promote metformin to healthy people who want to reduce their risk of cancer, diabetes, vascular occlusion, and obesity. This fatal departure from reality continues unabated, as our dysfunctional political/legal system denies information about metformin that could spare countless numbers of lives.

Type II diabetics suffer sharply higher rates of cancer[4-7] and vascular disease.[8-11] The anti-diabetic drug metformin has been shown in numerous scientific studies to slash the risk of cancer[12-24] and lower markers of vascular disease.[25-28] Metformin was shown to reduce blood sugar levels in the 1920s.[28] One reason it fell off the radar screen is that insulin quickly became popular because it produced an immediate glucose-lowering effect. What doctors back then did not realize is that while insulin saved the lives of type I diabetics (who produce little or no insulin), those with type II diabetes often produce too much insulin as their pancreas tries to offset multiple metabolic imbalances.

One of the metabolic imbalances of type II diabetes is the excess formation of glucose in the liver. To ensure that blood glucose never drops too low, the liver manufactures glucose in a process called gluconeogenesis. In type II diabetes, despite an elevated blood glucose level, the liver inappropriately continues to pump out glucose. This inappropriate outburst of glucose from the liver in type II diabetes patients is a classic hallmark of the disease. In fact, scientific data that measures glucose output by the liver shows that the typical type II diabetic produces three times more glucose in their liver than non-diabetics.[29] And, as we have previously reported, even most non-diabetics produce too much glucose in their liver as they age.

Scientific data shows that metformin reduces glucose production and the rate of gluconeogenesis by anywhere from 24% to 36%, respectively, thus reducing blood glucose levels while lowering the amount of insulin that is chronically secreted.[29] Metformin also enhances insulin sensitivity, thus enabling cells to remove more glucose from the bloodstream, which further lowers glucose and insulin levels.[30-33] In a study conducted by a team of researchers in Italy, 500 mg three times a day of metformin reduced insulin levels by 25%.

EXCESS INSULIN IS A "DEATH HORMONE"

In response to continuous over-production of glucose by the liver, the pancreas secretes huge amounts of insulin to suppress it. This excess amount of insulin damages blood vessel walls[34-36] and promotes tumor growth.[37-41] For a type II diabetic who is over-producing insulin, the use of insulin injections provides a relatively brief respite from high blood glucose levels—with horrific long-term consequences. Drug companies today are heavily promoting convenient insulin injection devices to physicians and suggesting that many of them have forgotten about insulin's proven glucose-lowering effects. The harsh reality is that for most type II diabetics, excess insulin represents a "death hormone" that causes weight gain,[42-44] cancer,[45-47] and vascular disease.[48-51]

It was not only the discovery of insulin that delayed recognition of metformin. Drugs known as sulfonylureas promote the insulin release from the pancreas. Sulfonylureas were liberally prescribed for decades and are another ill-conceived way of temporarily suppressing blood glucose at the expense of systemic metabolic havoc. Like insulin, sulfonylurea drugs induce weight gain, which is the opposite effect one is seeking when treating most type II diabetics. All sulfonylureas carry an FDA-mandated warning about increased risk of cardiovascular death.

In one study lasting more than 10 years, patients who primarily received metformin had a 39% reduction in the risk of heart attack and a 36% reduction of death from any cause.[52] The same study showed that metformin did not cause weight gain in overweight patients, while patients prescribed sulfonylureas gained more than 7 pounds, and those using insulin injections gained over 10 pounds.[53] For the multi-decade period Americans were denied access to metformin, doctors felt they had little choice but to prescribe sulfonylurea drugs and insulin injections. The needless suffering and death endured by diabetics during this "dark age" of American medicine is incalculable.

WHY AMERICAN DOCTORS WERE AFRAID OF METFORMIN

For decades, the American medical establishment labored under an egregious misconception about the safety of metformin. The reason was that drugs in the same class of metformin (biguanides) can cause a potentially fatal condition called lactic acidosis, where the body becomes overly acidic in the presence of excess lactic acid. While other biguanide drugs were withdrawn because of lactic acidosis risk, it turned out that metformin did not induce this same side effect in healthier people.[54] As long as one has sufficient kidney, liver, cardiac, and pulmonary function, any excess lactic acid caused by metformin is safely removed by the kidneys.[55-57] It turned out that only patients with severe kidney, liver, pulmonary, or cardiac impairment had to avoid metformin because of lactic acidosis concerns, and even these worries were overblown.

I'll never forget what a brilliant medical doctor personally told me after a large study came out that dispelled the myth connecting metformin with lactic acidosis. This doctor knew how effective metformin was, but was terrified of creating lactic acidosis in any of his patients. He told me something to the effect of, "If this study showing lactic acidosis is not a risk for metformin users is true, then the multi-decade oversight that caused doctors to fear metformin represents one of the great blunders in medical history."

The regrettable fact is that doctors in the United States were taught to avoid drugs in the class of metformin, even though metformin itself was being safely used throughout the world. If only the medical establishment in the United States had looked across the border as close as Canada, they would have seen metformin being liberally prescribed without the incidences of lactic acidosis they feared.

In the early years, when I was taking metformin for anti-aging purposes, most doctors warned me about lactic acidosis risk. I always asked where in the scientific literature does it show a healthy person is at risk for lactic acidosis when taking metformin? They could never cite a reference, so I continued taking my metformin.

ANALYSIS SHOWS METFORMIN DOES NOT CAUSE LACTIC ACIDOSIS

A Cochrane Systematic Review of over 300 trials evaluated the incidence of lactic acidosis among patients prescribed metformin vs. non-metformin anti-diabetes medications. Of 100,000 people, the incidence of lactic acidosis was 4.3 cases in the metformin group and 5.4

cases in the non-metformin group. The authors concluded that metformin is not associated with an increased risk for lactic acidosis.[58]

HOW METFORMIN FUNCTIONS

Metformin reduces blood glucose levels primarily by suppressing glucose formation in the liver (hepatic gluconeogenesis).[59] More importantly, it activates an enzyme called AMPK (AMP-activated protein kinase) that plays an important role in insulin signaling, systemic energy balance, and the metabolism of glucose and fats.[60] Activation of AMPK is one mechanism that may explain why diabetics prescribed metformin have sharply lower cancer rates. For instance, in a controlled study at MD Anderson Cancer Center, the risk of pancreatic cancer was 62% lower in diabetics who had taken metformin compared to those who had never taken it.[61] Diabetics suffer sharply higher incidences of pancreatic cancer than non-diabetics.[61]

YOUR NUTRIENTS "MAY" WORK AS WELL AS METFORMIN

Virtually every Life Extension® client takes curcumin on a daily basis. Curcumin activates the same AMPK enzyme at a rate that may be higher than metformin. Curcumin also increases insulin sensitivity while reducing expression of glucose-producing genes.[80] Coffee rich in chlorogenic acid has demonstrated a profound reduction in gluconeogenesis—with a corresponding decrease in post-meal glucose elevations.[81-83]

We know that suppression of gluconeogenesis, enhanced insulin sensitivity, and activation of AMPK are some of the mechanisms behind metformin's broad-spectrum benefits. It is not possible at this time, however, to know for sure if aging humans can derive identical benefits from nutrients like curcumin and chlorogenic acid as are provided by metformin. With my understanding of the beneficial mechanisms of curcumin and chlorogenic acid, I personally take these nutrients plus a high dose (850 mg) of metformin two to three times a day.

HOW METFORMIN MAY INCREASE HEART ATTACK RISK

Metformin reduces triglycerides,[62-64] glucose,[32,65,66] insulin,[67-69] and hemoglobin A1C (a marker of long-term glucose control).[32,70] These blood markers are all proven heart attack risk factors. Yet not all studies show metformin reduces heart attack incidence. One study found that when metformin was added to a group of non-overweight patients taking sulfonylurea drugs, there was a significant increase in overall mortality.[71] This suggests that metformin should not be combined with sulfonylureas. Furthermore, not all studies show that metformin reduces cardiovascular risk or improves overall survival in type II diabetic patients. There are several reasons to explain these discrepancies.

Metformin is known to cause vitamin B12 deficiency which translates into higher levels of artery-clogging homocysteine.[72-74] The tiny amount of vitamin B12 and other B-vitamins found in commercial supplements is not always sufficient to offset this problem. Those who take metformin should ensure they are taking higher doses of B-vitamins (at least 300 mcg of vitamin B12) and check their homocysteine levels to make sure it stays in the safer ranges.[75] One study showed that the addition of 5,000 mcg of folic acid to patients taking metformin reduced their homocysteine from 15.1 μmol/L to 12.1 μmol/L. Optimal homocysteine levels are probably under 8 μmol/L, but any reduction is helpful. Sadly, most diabetics prescribed metformin don't check their homocysteine levels and don't take enough B-vitamins to prevent a deficiency.

Some studies show that metformin reduces free testosterone and total testosterone levels in men.[77] Testosterone is especially important in male diabetics as it significantly enhances insulin sensitivity.[78] Life Extension® has previously published clinical data showing the critical importance of diabetic men to maintain youthful testosterone levels in order to improve glucose utilization.[79]

The greatest challenge in evaluating clinical data on metformin is that it is often prescribed to debilitated patients who have undergone severe arterial attack for many decades. These diabetic patients are at significant risk of cardiovascular disease from a number of underlying causes. They need to take aggressive steps to correct all independent risk factors for vascular disease, something that is never done in clinical studies.

POLITICIANS OVERLOOK MOST IMPORTANT ISSUE

Billions of dollars are being spent on campaign ads by politicians. Most of the issues raised will not directly affect you in a meaningful way. Overlooked is a problem that will affect every one of us—the suffocating impact of antiquated legislation on medical progress. Once you or a family member is diagnosed with a disease like pancreatic cancer, campaign ads become background clutter. Your only concern is finding a therapy that offers some hope of survival.

The best our current archaic system offers for pancreatic cancer is a drug called gemcitabine. Compared to another chemo drug, gemcitabine increased average survival by a meager 36 days, which conventional doctors described as a "significant improvement."[91] A team of researchers was able to improve on gemcitabine by using instead a toxic combination of chemotherapy drugs (called FOLFIRINOX). Compared to the gemcitabine group, patients able to tolerate the debilitating side effects of FOLFIRINOX lived 4.3 months longer than the gemcitabine group, but suffered greater toxicity.[92,93]

The fact that pancreatic cancer still quickly kills virtually everyone who contracts it is a stark example of how today's regulatory system stifles innovation. Unregulated environments have produced technologies like hand-held computers (smartphones) that perform miraculously and are affordable to mostly everyone. Life Extension® for years has provided hard-core scientific documentation about the anti-cancer properties of metformin. Yet unless the current political/legal stranglehold over medical innovation is lifted, the only cancer patients likely to benefit from metformin will be readers of *Life Extension Magazine* who insist their doctors prescribe it. Recall that metformin was discovered 90 years ago, yet conventional doctors are still failing to use it in the prevention and treatment of a host of age-related disorders.

SHOULD YOU ASK YOUR DOCTOR ABOUT METFORMIN?

Metformin is a synthetic compound available in low cost generic form. The challenge many people face is persuading their doctors to prescribe metformin if they are not diabetic. You may recall the many articles we have published showing that any elevation of fasting glucose above 85 mg/dL increases one's risk for contracting classic diabetic complications like heart attack and stroke.[84-90] Therefore, those whose glucose levels exceed 85 mg/dL should consider metformin for its glucose-lowering properties alone, though there are nutrients that may accomplish a similar effect.

No one should take metformin without having a complete battery of blood tests to show their doctor that it is not contraindicated because of disorders like kidney failure. Those with low blood sugar (hypoglycemia) may not be able to use metformin. A suggested starting dose of metformin is 250 mg before a large meal. The dose may be increased after a week to 250 mg before three meals a day. After a month, you may consider increasing to 500 mg before meals and eventually go up to 850 mg before meals, which is the upper limit dose. If you notice a slight reduction in appetite, use it to cut back on your calorie intake and hopefully shed some fat pounds. By stabilizing blood sugar and insulin levels, metformin can help reduce food cravings.

THE POLITICAL/LEGAL SYSTEM MUST BE CHANGED

Human clinical research has long been oppressed in the United States by a variety of laws that conspire to deny medical progress. The few new therapies that are approved are mediocre, expensive, and often laden with side effects. The current system represents the worst of all worlds when it comes to the kind of scientific advances that aging people need to significantly extend their healthy life spans.

Your support of Life Extension® enables us to continue our relentless campaign to tear down the strangleholds erected by public and private institutions. The 37-year delay in approving metformin provides a real-world example of how broken our political/legal systems are when it comes to finding cures for degenerative disease and the aging process itself.

WHAT YOU CAN DO TO STOP NEEDLESS SUFFERING AND DEATH

Scientists have identified novel ways of treating cancer and other illnesses, but too little of this new technology is being used in clinical practice. When new discoveries are made, drug companies spend years seeking a patent, and then more years carrying it through the cumbersome bureaucratic approval process. A major reason so many cancer patients die today is an antiquated regulatory system that causes effective therapies to be delayed (or suppressed altogether).

This system must be changed, if the 1,500 American cancer patients who perish each day are to have a realistic chance of being saved. Our long-standing proposal has been to change the law so that anyone can opt out of the FDA's umbrella of "protection." This approach will allow companies to sell drugs that have demonstrated safety and a reasonable likelihood of effectiveness, which are clearly labeled "Not Approved by the FDA." Patients who wish can still use only FDA-approved drugs, while those willing to take a risk, in consultation with their doctors, will be allowed to try drugs shown to be safe that are still not approved.

We believe that this initiative will result in a renaissance in the practice of medicine similar to the computer technology revolution of the past four decades. In this environment, many lethal diseases will succumb to cures that are less expensive than is presently the case. And greater competition will help eliminate the healthcare cost crisis that exists today. Seriously ill people, in consultation with their doctors, should be able to make up their own minds about what drugs they are willing to try.

This is the time when political leaders will at least listen to their constituent's concerns. I encourage each of you to log on to our legislative action website at www.lef.org/lac to easily email your Representative and two Senators a letter demanding they enact legislation that will enable those with serious illness to obtain therapies far enough along in the clinical trials process to be deemed safe, but not yet approved by the FDA.

TAKE ACTION NOW!
Tell Congress to Change the Law!

There are millions of cancer patients alive right now who face possible or probable death in the next twelve months. If you add their family members and friends, there are tens of millions of Americans who should be outraged by an outdated regulatory system that bans access to potentially life-saving therapies.

The FDA continues to suppress innovative therapies because the public has failed to demand that our elected officials rein in the FDA's arbitrary authority. The first step in changing today's outmoded system is for those who understand the magnitude of this problem to communicate the urgent need for change to Congress. Those concerned about this serious issue should log on to www. lef.org/lac to insist that their Representative and two Senators help enact legislation that will enable cancer patients to obtain therapies far enough along in the clinical trials process to be deemed safe, but not yet approved by the FDA.

Take Action Now!

In addition to logging on to www.lef.org/lac to write your members of Congress, I also ask that you phone your Congressional members at 1-202-224-3121 to let them know how disgusted you are that doctors and patients are not allowed to choose drugs that may be effective against an often fatal disease.

Here is a phone script you can use when speaking to legislative staff members:

> I ask that you sponsor or co-sponsor legislation to enable cancer patients (and those with other serious diseases) to purchase medications while they are pending final approval by the FDA. This approach will allow companies to sell novel drugs with a label clearly stating that they are "Not Approved by the FDA."

> Consumers who wish to rely on the FDA can limit their choices to fully approved drugs only, while those willing to take a risk (in consultation with their doctors) will be allowed to try what they choose. (Companies that make fraudulent claims for products can be prosecuted under the laws that exist today.)

> This initiative can result in a renaissance in the practice of medicine, similar to the computer technology revolution that has occurred over the past three decades. In this environment free of regulatory burden, many inexpensive cures will very likely be found for lethal diseases. And greater competition will help eliminate the healthcare cost crisis that exists today.

> I am tired of reading about medical breakthroughs, only to be told that I will have to wait years before the therapy might become available. As 1,500 Americans die of cancer each day, I consider the introduction and passage of such a law an extremely high priority.

Seriously ill people have the fundamental right to make up their own minds about what drugs they are allowed to try, in consultation with their physicians. Please let me know that you will sponsor or co-sponsor such legislation, which will provide us with quicker access to drugs that the FDA has found safe and potentially effective, but have not yet received final approval.

References

1. Available at: http://onlinelibrary.wiley.com/doi/10.1111/j.1464-5491.2011.03469.x/pdf. Accessed August 2, 2012.
2. Available at: http://www.lef.org/magazine/mag96/sept96_freedom.html. Accessed May 11, 2012.
3. Available at: http://www.cnn.com/2012/04/05/health/diabetes-drug-fights-cancer/. Accessed May 11, 2012.
4. Castillo JJ, Mull N, Reagan JL, Nemr S, Mitri J. Increased incidence of non-Hodgkin lymphoma, leukemia, and myeloma in patients with diabetes mellitus type 2: a meta-analysis of observational studies. *Blood*. 2012 May 24;119(21):4845–50.
5. Vigneri P, Frasca F, Sciacca L, Pandini G, Vigneri R. Diabetes and cancer. *Endocr Relat Cancer*. 2009 Dec;16(4):1103–23.
6. Michels KB, Solomon CG, Hu FB, et al. Type II diabetes and subsequent incidence of breast cancer in the Nurses' Health Study. *Diabetes Care*. 2003 Jun;26(6):1752–8.
7. Aschebrook-Kilfoy B, Sabra MM, Brenner A, et al. Diabetes and thyroid cancer risk in the National Institutes of Health-AARP Diet and Health Study. *Thyroid*. 2011 Sep;21(9):957–63.
8. Haffner SM, Miettinen H. Insulin resistance implications for type II diabetes mellitus and coronary heart disease. *Am J Med*. 1997 Aug;103(2):152–62.
9. Mazzone T, Chait A, Plutzky J. Cardiovascular disease risk in type 2 diabetes mellitus: insights from mechanistic studies. *Lancet*. 2008 May 24;371(9626):1800–9.

10. Alexander CM, Landsman PB, Teutsch SM, Haffner SM. Third National Health and Nutrition Examination Survey (NHANES III); National Cholesterol Education Program (NCEP). NCEP-defined metabolic syndrome, diabetes, and prevalence of coronary heart disease among NHANES III participants age 50 years and older. *Diabetes.* 2003 May;52(5): 1210–4.

11. Schurgin S, Rich S, Mazzone T. Increased prevalence of significant coronary artery calcification in patients with diabetes. *Diabetes Care.* 2001 Feb;24(2):335–8.

12. Libby G, Donnelly LA, Donnan PT, Alessi DR, Morris AD, Evans JM. New users of metformin are at low risk of incident cancer: a cohort study among people with type 2 diabetes. *Diabetes Care.* 2009 Sep;32(9):1620–5.

13. Romero IL, McCormick A, McEwen KA, et al. Relationship of type II diabetes and metformin use to ovarian cancer progression, survival, and chemosensitivity. *Obstet Gynecol.* 2012 Jan;119(1):61–7.

14. Li D, Yeung SC, Hassan MM, Konopleva M, Abbruzzese JL. Antidiabetic therapies affect risk of pancreatic cancer. *Gastroenterology.* 2009 Aug;137(2):482–8.

15. Wang LW, Li ZS, Zou DW, Jin ZD, Gao J, Xu GM. Metformin induces apoptosis of pancreatic cancer cells. *World J Gastroenterol.* 2008 Dec 21;14(47):7192–8.

16. Wright JL, Stanford JL. Metformin use and prostate cancer in Caucasian men: results from a population-based case-control study. *Cancer Causes Control.* 2009 Nov;20(9):1617–22.

17. Bodmer M, Meier C, Krahenbuhl S, Jick SS, Meier CR. Long-term metformin use is associated with decreased risk of breast cancer. *Diabetes Care.* 2010 Jun;33(6):1304–8.

18. Cantrell LA, Zhou C, Mendivil A, Malloy KM, Gehrig PA, Bae-Jump VL. Metformin is a potent inhibitor of endometrial cancer cell proliferation—implications for a novel treatment strategy. *Gynecol Oncol.* 2010 Jan;116(1):92–8.

19. Hirsch HA, Iliopoulos D, Tsichlis PN, Struhl K. Metformin selectively targets cancer stem cells, and acts together with chemotherapy to block tumor growth and prolong remission. *Cancer Res.* 2009 Oct 1;69(19):7507–11.

20. Anisimov VN, Egormin PA, Piskunova TS, et al. Metformin extends life span of HER-2/neu transgenic mice and in combination with melatonin inhibits growth of transplantable tumors in vivo. *Cell Cycle.* 2010 Jan 1;9(1):188–97.

21. Evans JM, Donnelly LA, Emslie-Smith AM, Alessi DR, Morris AD. Metformin and reduced risk of cancer in diabetic patients. *BMJ.* 2005 Jun 4;330(7503):1304–5.

22. Hosono K, Endo H, Takahashi H, et al. Metformin suppresses colorectal aberrant crypt foci in a short-term clinical trial. *Cancer Prev Res (Phila).* 2010 Sep;3(9):1077–83.

23. Onitilo AA, Engel JM, Glurich I, Stankowski RV, Williams GM, Doi SA. Diabetes and cancer II: role of diabetes medications and influence of shared risk factors. *Cancer Causes Control.* 2012 Jul;23(7):991–1008. Epub 2012 Apr 25.

24. Memmott RM, Mercado JR, Maier CR, Kawabata S, Fox SD, Dennis PA. Metformin prevents tobacco carcinogen-induced lung tumorigenesis. *Cancer Prev Res (Phila).* 2010 Sep;3(9):1066–76.

25. Nagi DK, Yudkin JS. Effects of metformin on insulin resistance, risk factors for cardiovascular disease, and plasminogen activator inhibitor in NIDDM subjects. A study of two ethnic groups. *Diabetes Care.* 1993 16(4):621–29.

26. Evans JM, Ogston SA, Emslie-Smith A, Morris AD. Risk of mortality and adverse cardiovascular outcomes in type 2 diabetes: a comparison of patients treated with sulfonylureas and metformin. *Diabetologia.* 2006 May;49(5):930–6.

27. Brame L, Verma S, Anderson T, Lteif A, Mather K. Insulin resistance as a therapeutic target for improved endothelial function: metformin. *Curr Drug Targets Cardiovasc Haematol Disord.* 2004 Mar;4(1):53–63.

28. Available at: http://www.idb.hr/diabetologia/10no3-2.pdf. Accessed August 2, 2012.

29. Hundal RS, Krssak M, Dufour S, et al. Mechanism by which metformin reduces glucose production in type 2 diabetes. *Diabetes*. 2000 Dec;49(12):2063–9.

30. Moon RJ. The addition of metformin in type 1 diabetes improves insulin sensitivity, diabetic control, body composition and patient well-being. *Diabetes Obes Metab*. 2007 Jan;9(1):143–5.

31. Wong AK, Symon R, Alzadjali MA, et al. The effect of metformin on insulin resistance and exercise parameters in patients with heart failure. *Eur J Heart Fail*. 2012 Jun 27. [Epub ahead of print]

32. Boyda HN, Procyshyn RM, Tse L, et al. Differential effects of 3 classes of antidiabetic drugs on olanzapine-induced glucose dysregulation and insulin resistance in female rats. *J Psychiatry Neurosci*. 2012 May 28;37(4):110140. doi: 10.1503/jpn.110140. [Epub ahead of print]

33. Campagnoli C, Pasanisi P, Abbà C, et al. Effect of different doses of metformin on serum testosterone and insulin in non-diabetic women with breast cancer: a randomized study. *Clin Breast Cancer*. 2012 Jun;12(3):175–82.

34. Cersosimo E, DeFronzo RA. Insulin resistance and endothelial dysfunction: the road map to cardiovascular diseases. *Diabetes Metab Res Rev*. 2006 Nov-Dec;22(6):423–36.

35. Eschwège E. The dysmetabolic syndrome, insulin resistance and increased cardiovascular (CV) morbidity and mortality in type 2 diabetes: aetiological factors in the development of CV complications. *Diabetes Metab*. 2003 Sep;29(4 Pt 2):6S19–27.

36. Osei K. Insulin resistance and systemic hypertension. *Am J Cardiol*. 1999 Jul 8;84(1A):33J-36J.

37. Tran TT, Medline A, Bruce WR. Insulin promotion of colon tumors in rats. *Cancer Epidemiol Biomarkers Prev*. 1996 Dec;5(12):1013–5.

38. Parekh N, Lin Y, Hayes RB, Albu JB, Lu-Yao GL. Longitudinal associations of blood markers of insulin and glucose metabolism and cancer mortality in the T hird National Health and Nutrition Examination Survey. *Cancer Causes Control.* 2010 Apr;21(4):631–42.

39. Otani T, Iwasaki M, Sasazuki S, Inoue M, Tsugane S; Japan Public Health Center-based Prospective Study Group. Plasma C-peptide, insulin-like growth factor-I, insulin-like growth factor binding proteins and risk of colorectal cancer in a nested case-control study: the Japan public health center-based prospective study. *Int J Cancer.* 2007 May 1;120(9):2007–12.

40. Ma J, Li H, Giovannucci E, et al. Prediagnostic body-mass index, plasma C-peptide concentration, and prostate cancer-specific mortality in men with prostate cancer: a long-term survival analysis. *Lancet Oncol.* 2008 Nov;9(11):1039–47.

41. Hirose K, Toyama T, Iwata H, Takezaki T, Hamajima N, Tajima K. Insulin, insulin-like growth factor-I and breast cancer risk in Japanese women. *Asian Pac J Cancer Prev.* 2003 Jul-Sep;4(3):239–46.

42. Sigal RJ, El-Hashimy M, Martin BC, Soeldner JS, Krolewski AS, Warram JH. Acute postchallenge hyperinsulinemia predicts weight gain: a prospective study. *Diabetes.* 1997 Jun;46(6):1025–9.

43. Russell-Jones D, Khan R. Insulin-associated weight gain in diabetes—causes, effects and coping strategies. *Diabetes Obes Metab.* 2007 Nov;9(6):799–812.

44. Johnson MS, Figueroa-Colon R, Huang TT, Dwyer JH, Goran MI. Longitudinal changes in body fat in African-American and caucasian children: influence of fasting insulin and insulin sensitivity. *J Clin Endocrinol Metab.* 2001 Jul;86(7):3182–7.

45. Bowker SL, Majumdar SR, Veugelers P, Johnson JA. Increased cancer-related mortality for patients with type

2 diabetes who use sulfonylureas or insulin. *Diabetes Care* 2006 Feb;29(2):254–8.

46. Kaaks R. Plasma insulin, IGF-I and breast cancer. *Gynecol Obstet Fertil*. 2001 Mar;29(3):185–91.

47. Nilsen TI, Vatten LJ. Prospective study of colorectal cancer risk and physical activity, diabetes, blood glucose and BMI: exploring the hyperinsulinaemia hypothesis. *Br J Cancer*. 2001 Feb 2;84(3): 417–22.

48. Hegele RA. Premature atherosclerosis associated with monogenic insulin resistance. *Circulation*. 2001 May 8;103(18):2225–9.

49. Chu N, Spiegelman D, Hotamisligil GS, Rifai N, Stampler M, Rimm EB. Plasma insulin, leptin, and soluble TNF receptors levels in relation to obesity-related atherogenic and thrombogenic cardiovascular disease risk factors among men. *Atherosclerosis*. 2001 Aug;157(2):495–503.

50. Lichtenstein MJ, Yarnell JW, Elwood PC, et al. Sex hormones, insulin, lipids, and prevalent ischemic heart disease. *Am J Epidemiol*. 1987 Oct;126(4):647–57.

51. Dekker JM, Girman C, Rhodes T, et al. Metabolic syndrome and 10-year cardio-vascular disease risk in the Hoorn Study. *Circulation*. 2005 Aug 2;112(5):666–73.

52. Available at: http://www.nejm.org/doi/full/10.1056/NEJMoa0806470#t=article. Accessed July 11, 2012.

53. Available at: http://www.bmj.com/content/310/6972/83.full. Accessed July 11, 2012.

54. Available at: http://www.medscape.com/viewarticle/714920. Accessed July 11, 2012.

55. Klow NE, Draganov B, Os I. Metformin and contrast media-increased risk of lactic acidosis. *Tidsskr Nor Laegeforen*. 2001 Jun 10;121(15):1829.

56. Brown JB, Pedula K, Barzilay J, Herson MK, Latare P. Lactic acidosis rates in typeII diabetes. *Diabetes Care*. 1998 Oct;21(10):1659–63.

57. Misbin RI. The phantom of lactic acidosis due to metformin in patients with diabetes. *Diabetes Care*. 2004 Jul;27(7): 1791–3.

58. Salpeter S, Greyber E, Pasternak G, Salpeter E. Risk of fatal and nonfatal lactic acidosis with metformin use in type 2 diabetes mellitus. *Cochrane Database Syst Rev*. 2010 Apr 14;(4):CD002967.

59. Kirpichnikov D, McFarlane SI, Sowers JR. Metformin: an update. *Ann Intern Med*. 2002 137(1):25–33.

60. Towler MC, Hardie DG. AMP-activated protein kinase in metabolic control and insulin signaling. *Circ Res*. 2007 100(3):328–41.

61. Li D, Yeung SC, Hassan MM, Konopleva M, Abbruzzese JL. Antidiabetic therapies affect risk of pancreatic cancer. *Gastroenterology*. 2009 Aug;137(2):482–8.

62. Emral R, Köseoğlulari O, Tonyukuk V, Uysal AR, Kamel N, Corapçioğlu D. The effect of short-term glycemic regulation with gliclazide and metformin on postprandial lipemia. *Exp Clin Endocrinol Diabetes*. 2005 Feb;113(2):80–4.

63. Mughal MA, Jan M, Maheri WM, Memon MY, Ali M. The effect of metformin on glycemic control, serum lipids and lipoproteins in diet alone and sulfonylurea-treated type 2 diabetic patients with sub-optimal metabolic control. *J Pak Med Assoc*. 2000 Nov;50(11):381–6.

64. Lund SS, Tarnow L, Frandsen M, et al. Impact of metformin versus the prandial insulin secretagogue, repaglinide, on fasting and postprandial glucose and lipid responses in non-obese patients with type 2 diabetes. *Eur J Endocrinol*. 2008 Jan;158(1):35–46.

65. Hundal RS, Krssak M, Dufour S, et al. Mechanism by which metformin reduces glucose production in type 2 diabetes. *Diabetes*. 2000 Dec;49(12):2063–9.

66. Bjørnholt JV, Erikssen G, Aaser E, et al. Fasting blood glucose: an underestimated risk factor for cardiovascular death.

Results from a 22-year follow-up of healthy nondiabetic men. *Diabetes Care.* 1999 Jan;22(1):45–9.

67. Goodwin PJ, Pritchard KI, Ennis M, Clemons M, Graham M, Fantus IG. Insulin-lowering effects of metformin in women with early breast cancer. *Clin Breast Cancer.* 2008 Dec;8(6):501–5.

68. Velazquez EM, Mendosa S, Hamer T, Sosa F, Glucck CJ. Metformin therapy in women with polycystic ovary syndrome reduces hyperinsulinemia, insulin resistance, hyperandrogenemia, and systolic blood pressure, while facilitating menstrual regularity and pregnancy. *Metabolism.* 1994 May;43(5):647–54.

69. MB Davidson, AL Peters. An overview of metformin in the treatment of type 2 diabetes mellitus. *Am J Med.* 1997Jan;102(1):99–110.

70. Avilés-Santa L, Sinding J, Raskin P. Effects of metformin in patients with poorly controlled, insulin-treated type 2 diabetes mellitus. A randomized, double-blind, placebo-controlled trial. *Ann Intern Med.* 1999 Aug 3;131(3):182–8.

71. Olsson J, Lindberg G, Gottsäter M, et al. Increased mortality in Type II diabetic patients using sulphonylurea and metformin in combination: a population-based observational study. *Diabetologia.* 2000 May;43(5):558–60.

72. Mazokopakis EE, Starakis IK. Recommendations for diagnosis and management of metformin-induced vitamin B12 (Cbl)deficiency. *Diabetes Res Clin Pract.* 2012 Jul 7. [Epub ahead of print]

73. Carlsen SM, Følling I, Grill V, Bjerve KS, Schneede J, Refsum H. Metformin increases total serum homocysteine levels in non-diabetic male patients with coronary heart disease. *Scand J Clin Lab Invest.* 1997 Oct;57(6):521–7.

74. de Jager J, Kooy A, Lehert P, et al. Long term treatment with metformin in patients with type 2 diabetes and risk of vitamin

B-12 deficiency: randomised placebo controlled trial. *BMJ*. 2010 May 20;340:c2181. doi: 10.1136/bmj.c2181.

75. Langan RC, Zawistoski KJ. Update on vitamin B12 deficiency. *Am Fam Physician*. 2011 Jun 15;83(12):1425–30.

76. Aghamohammadi V, Gargari BP, Aliasgharzadeh A. Effect of folic acid supplementation on homocysteine, serum total antioxidant capacity, and malondialdehyde in patients with type 2 diabetes mellitus. *J Am Coll Nutr*. 2011 Jun;30(3):210–5.

77. Ozata M, Oktenli C, Bingol N, Ozdemir IC. The effects of metformin and diet on plasma testosterone and leptin levels in obese men. *Obes Res*. 2001 Nov;9(11):662–7.

78. Grossmann M, Thomas MC, Panagiotopoulos S, et al. Low testosterone levels are common and associated with insulin resistance in men with diabetes. *J Clin Endocrinol Metab*. 2008 May;93(5): 1834–40.

79. Available at:http://www.lef.org/magazine/mag2007/jul2007_report_diabetes_01.htm. Accessed July 9, 2012.

80. Kim T, Davis J, Zhang AJ, He X, Mathews ST. Curcumin activates AMPK and suppresses gluconeogenic gene expression in hepatoma cells. *Biochem Biophys Res Commun*. 2009 Oct 16;388(2):377–82.

81. Henry-Vitrac C, Ibarra A, Roller M, Merillon JM, Vitrac X. Contribution of chlorogenic acids to the inhibition of human hepatic glucose-6-phosphatase activity in vitro by Svetol, a standardized decaffeinated green coffee extract. *J Agric Food Chem*. 2010 Apr 14;58(7):4141–4.

82. Andrade-Cetto A, Vazquez RC. Gluconeogenesis inhibition and phytochemical composition of two Cecropia species. *J Ethnopharmacol*. 2010 Jul 6;130(1):93–7.

83. Nagendran MV. Effect of Green Coffee Bean Extract (GCE), High in Chlorogenic Acids, on Glucose Metabolism. Poster presentation number: 45-LB-P. Obesity 2011, the 29th Annual Scientific Meeting of the Obesity Society. Orlando, Florida. October 1–5, 2011.

84. Available at: http://www.lef.org/magazine/mag2012/feb2012_Doctors-Overlook-Leading-Cause-Premature-Death_01.htm. Accessed July 11,2012.

85. Available at: http://www.lef.org/magazine/mag2012/feb2012_Suppress-Deadly-After-Meal-Blood-Sugar-Surges_01.htm. Accessed July 11, 2012.

86. Available at: http://www.lef.org/magazine/mag2011/ss2011_Are-We-All-Pre-Diabetic_01.htm. Accessed July 11, 2012.

87. Available at: http://www.lef.org/magazine/mag2011/ss2011_Effective-Approaches-to-Blunt-Blood-Sugar-Surges_01.htm. Accessed July 11, 2012.

88. Available at: http://www.lef.org/magazine/mag2011/jan2011_Glucose-The-Silent-Killer_01.htm. Accessed July 11, 2012.

89. Available at: http://www.lef.org/magazine/mag2010/ss2010_Protect-Your-Body-from-a-Silent-Killer_01.htm. Accessed July 11, 2012.

90. Available at: http://www.lef.org/magazine/mag2004/jan2004_awsi_01.htm. Accessed July 11, 2012.

91. Burris HA III, Moore MJ, Andersen J, et al. Improvements in survival and clinical benefit with gemcitabine as first-line therapy for patients with advanced pancreas cancer: a randomized trial. *J Clin Oncol*. 1997 Jun;15(6):2403–13.

92. Conroy T, Desseigne F, Ychou M, et al. FOLFIRINOX versus gemcitabine for metastatic pancreatic cancer. *N Engl J Med*. 2011 May 12;364(19):1817–25.

93. Lowery MA, O'Reilly EM. Genomics and pharmacogenomics of pancreatic adenocarcinoma. *Pharmacogenomics J*. 2012 Feb;12(1):1–9.

Big Pharma: Putting Profits above Patients

Large pharmaceutical companies today wield enormous power. These giants of the medical industry spend vast sums on research and development of new drugs and reap hundreds of billions of dollars in sales. Besides research outlays, Big Pharma funds a portion of the FDA budget, spends billions in lobbying Congress, and provides more campaign contributions than any other industry.* Does Big Pharma operate in the best interest of consumers and patients? If not, where is the watchdog to safeguard patients when health is threatened by harmful drugs? Who stands up for practitioners or innovators who develop competing treatments? In the next few chapters we provide a glimpse of the ruthless disregard for its own end users ruling the pharmaceutical industry.

---

* https://www.drugwatch.com/manufacturer/.

New England Journal of Medicine Exposes Generic Price Scandal

N O ONE HAS fought against high drug prices longer or harder than Life Extension®.[1-20] The penalty for exposing healthcare corruption is endless governmental investigations aimed at destroying our organization. The tide may be turning in our favor.

The *New England Journal of Medicine* published a report that uncovered a drug price scandal that we've sought to expose for the past four decades.[21] *CBS News* turned this consumer swindle into a headline report that graphically depicted the devastating impact that skyrocketing generic drug prices are having.[22] The next day, I gave an impromptu speech at an Alzheimer's seminar where I asked the audience to join me in amending the law to prohibit the FDA from granting monopoly status to generic drug makers.

Virtually everyone in the audience said they would personally take the time to protest high drug prices at local congressional offices.

Two months later, *60 Minutes* featured an in-depth report
on today's broken sick-care system. A quote from this *60
Minutes* broadcast relating to the Affordable Care Act
stated that it is the product of an " . . . orgy of lobbying
and backroom deals in which just about everyone with a
stake in the $3-trillion-a-year health industry came out
ahead—except the taxpayers." [23] The *60 Minutes* report
went on to state there is "no way in the world that we're
gonna be able to pay for it." Investigative journalists have
since corroborated how high drug prices are causing
American consumers to become serfs of the pharmaceutical industry.

Today's medical system provides mediocre efficacy at
prohibitive prices. When you read news stories about
municipal, corporate, or personal bankruptcies, the high
cost of healthcare is a consistent underlying factor. Misguided politicians believe that government subsidies,
mandates, and giveaways can resolve high sick-care costs.
Even a cursory glance at the extravagant prices of new
medications exposes the falsity of this charade. When
a single new drug can cost $100,000, and protocols are
being developed that combine several drugs priced in this
range, how can any form of "cost-sharing" be expected to
work? It has become mathematically impossible for these
outlandish sick-care costs to become "affordable" via government edict.

For example, a bottle of the prescription drug Valcyte®
contains 60 tablets. The price for this bottle of Valcyte®
is around $4,200. This works out to approximately $70 per
tablet. My cost for a four-month course of this medication is

over $16,000. Some people are spending over $50,000 a year for this drug to stay alive—and this is often just one of many medications they need. Before I describe a simple solution to this epidemic problem, I want to enlighten you to a growing scam in the prescription generic drug arena that finally is generating mainstream media coverage.

GENERIC DRUG PRICE GOUGING

Generic Drug	Price Increase per Pill	Percent Price Increase
Doxycycline (antibiotic)	6.3 cents to $3.36	5,300%
Captopril (antihypertensive)	1.4 cents to 39.9 cents	2,850%
Clomipramine (antidepressant)	22 cents to $8.32	3,780%

MAGNITUDE OF THE FRAUD

Price gouging on a growing number of generic drugs has grown beyond verbal description. In the box you see above are examples of price increases occurring in the generic drug marketplace reported on by the *New England Journal of Medicine*.[21] These kinds of price increases are not unique. They reflect a growing swath of generic drugs that cost virtually nothing to manufacture, but they are spiking to stratospheric consumer price levels.

The *New England Journal of Medicine* gave an example of a generic drug (albendazole) that costs less than one dollar per daily dose overseas, but has risen to $119 per typical daily dose in the United States ($3,570 per month). This is a 2,010% increase from what this same generic drug cost in 2010. Medicaid spending on this one drug alone (albendazole) spiked from $100,000 in 2008 to $7.5 million in 2013—a 75-fold increase![21]

WE'RE ALL BEING DEFRAUDED

Whether or not you need a generic drug whose price has exponentially increased, you are paying through higher health insurance premiums, higher deductibles, and higher co-pays, as well as limitations on what physician you may use and what services that doctor may perform. A generic drug that I use called tretinoin costs $1,100 per month. My health insurance covers $850, and I have to pick up the balance of $250 per month. This drug (tretinoin) was approved in 1995 and long ago lost patent protection, yet it is costing me $13,200 per year. I say me because I pay this extortionist price via my insurance premiums along with the many "exclusions" that cause me to pay out-of-pocket for what health insurance used to cover. What may shock you most is what the active ingredient of this drug costs. Consumers are paying over $1,100 for this bottle of tretinoin. Yet the active ingredient for the entire bottle costs a mere 80 cents. Even including encapsulation and quality control, that's a markup of about 400 times over the cost to make this off-patent drug.

As we reported in the September 2014 edition of *Life Extension Magazine®*, collusion among drug makers is causing generics to be priced beyond rational affordability.

The cover headline of the September 2014 issue was titled "How to Turn 8 Pennies Into $600." This was based on an article where I reveal that an antiviral cream (acyclovir) that long ago lost patent protection was being sold to pharmacies for 7,500% over the active ingredient cost. The active ingredient (acyclovir) costs only 8 pennies, yet pharmacies are paying a generic maker $600 for this drug and selling it to consumers for around $700.

The media has just started reporting on the magnitude of generic drug price gouging. These kinds of price markups are unsustainable. They are part of the reason why healthcare has become unaffordable whether or not you have so-called "insurance." An increasing number of experts are coming to this realization, including editors of the *New England Journal of Medicine* and other publications. We are all being defrauded by this unconscionable price gouging made possible by overregulation of prescription drugs.

I USED TO OWN A PHARMACY

I established a retail pharmacy (Life Extension Pharmacy®) in an attempt to slash the high cost of generic drugs. I was able to witness some of the manipulation going on behind the scenes that results in consumer prices for generics spiraling upward. Our pharmacists never knew what the price of a generic drug would be from day to day. Some drug companies "stop making" certain generics altogether, which usually results in a massive price spike from the remaining maker(s). This happens because competition has all but disappeared.

One reason I set up the Life Extension Pharmacy® in 2008 was to slash the prices of generic drugs to our members. Back then, pharmacies were selling generic drugs at out-of-pocket prices that were higher than what average people could afford. My goal of slashing consumer prescription drug costs was short-lived, as generic makers raised prices so high that even co-pays on certain drugs remained unaffordable, even though the cost to make most generics is virtually nothing.

THE POLITICIANS ARE CLUELESS

There has been more criticism leveled against the Affordable Care Act than perhaps any other piece of enacted legislation. Sound-bite-speaking political candidates constantly state that if elected they will "abolish it." The problem is none has the faintest clue what to replace it with. The reason they can't even pretend to have a solution is that none understands what's behind the healthcare cost crisis.

Do you think any politician today knows that there are generic drugs being sold for over $1,000 a month whose active ingredient costs only 80 cents? The politicians don't know this and it's hard to expect they would.

It is up to the citizenry to enlighten Congress and demand that the Food, Drug, and Cosmetic Act be amended so that free-market forces can quickly resolve this generic price-gouging scandal.

WHY THIS CONCERNS LIFE EXTENSION®

New readers may wonder why an organization like Life Extension®, which is best known for pioneering lifesaving nutrients like coenzyme Q10, is making a big deal about generic drug price gouging. One reason is that Life Extension® does far more than formulate advanced dietary supplements. Our *Disease Prevention and Treatment* protocols contain recommendations for people to ask their doctors about trying off-label drugs in order to achieve a better clinical outcome. Our track record of recommending off-label drugs like metformin and cimetidine to better treat disease is unparalleled.[24] Insurance companies, however, often refuse to pay for the off-label prescribed drugs we recommend.

If this price gouging does not stop, it will render off-label use of these drugs meaningless as consumers will not be able to afford the generic drug's high cost. So in addition to sparing this nation's sick-care system from economic collapse, we at Life Extension® need to ensure that affordable generic medications are available when the need arises for them.

A FREE-MARKET SOLUTION

The solution to this problem of rip-off drug pricing is to amend the Food, Drug, and Cosmetic Act to allow more competition in the generic marketplace. If enacted, generic prices will plummet to levels so low you won't even worry about what percentage your insurance company pays. When generic drugs drop this much, it will push down many patented pharmaceutical prices because generic substitutes often work as well as newer branded drugs.

Against us are pharmaceutical lobbyists who will do virtually anything to protect their lucrative monopoly against free-market competition. On our side are 330 million American consumers, most of whom cannot afford to fall ill even if they have health insurance. That's because the deductibles, co-pays, and exclusions result in enormous out-of-pocket expenses that are today's leading cause of personal bankruptcies. My question is how many of you want to take political action to stop this price gouging?

WE'VE FOUGHT THE DRUG CARTELS SINCE THE 1980s

Life Extension® learned about the rip-off prices Americans were paying for their medications in the 1980s. We launched a relentless campaign to educate the public and Congress about the high prices Americans were forced to pay compared to what identical medications cost in Europe and other countries. When digging through a box of old papers, I ran across one of the many newspaper ads our supporters paid for to expose the corrupt prices and drug approval delays that were killing American citizens. We've reproduced one of those ads from the year 1991 on the facing page.

You can see the date on this newspaper ad is October 11, 1991. On November 7, 1991, we were in handcuffs, standing before a federal judge, with the FDA insisting that we be denied bond because we represented a danger to the public (for informing Americans that lower-priced medications could be obtained almost anywhere else in the world). Fortunately, an avalanche of letters from our supporters to the judge helped persuade him to grant us bond ($1 million). The multiple charges the FDA tried to use to indict us were eventually dismissed by the Department of Justice in 1995–1996. If it were not for our supporters standing up to the FDA's attempts to incarcerate us, there would be no Life Extension® organization today, and supplements like coenzyme Q10 would likely be available only via expensive prescription.

Americans today routinely obtain lower-priced medications from Canada because they can access offshore pharmacies via the Internet. This was not the case in the 1980s–1990s. Back then, the FDA viciously fought anyone who dared to inform Americans where they could purchase less expensive medications.

LEGISLATION URGENTLY NEEDED!

Fighting the FDA's ban on personal use importations of medications was only one battle we spearheaded. The other dealt with the FDA's attempts to turn many dietary supplements into prescription drugs. When we initiated action to combat FDA's attempts to ban dietary supplements, a huge percentage of our supporters rallied to stop this from happening.

The result was passage of a bill (Dietary Supplement Health and Education Act-1994) that protected supplements and substantially lowered consumer prices.

MIAMI HERALD NEWSPAPER AD OUR SUPPORTERS PAID FOR TWENTY-SIX YEARS AGO—FRIDAY, OCTOBER 11, 1991

For those who think it's not worth the effort to let your voice be heard, consider the consequences of failing to take action. Seniors may have to return to the work force to afford their medications. Those working full time may have to find additional part-time work to pay the high premiums and many out-of-pocket expenses no longer covered by medical insurance. This problem can be partially resolved if free-market competition is allowed in the generic drug marketplace. If we can persuade Congress to amend the Food, Drug, and Cosmetic Act, the price of many generic drugs will plummet more than 90%.

We at Life Extension® are organizing a grassroots campaign to overwhelm the lobbyists that currently dominate Congress and the federal agencies that are adversely impacting our health and longevity. A website has been set up for those who want to enlist as activists to combat the atrocities perpetrated against the citizenry by our politicians and unelected/unaccountable bureaucrats. To enroll in this campaign to tear down high drug prices, log on to: LifeExtension.com/consumer.

FEEBLE SUGGESTIONS FROM THE AMERICAN MEDICAL ASSOCIATION

In recognition of the generic drug pricing scandal, the *Journal of the American Medical Association* (*JAMA*) published an editorial on November 24, 2015, titled "Options to Promote Competitive Generics Markets in the United States." Of interest was the citing of a statistic showing that 86% of all prescriptions written are for generic drugs. The editorial goes on to describe the problem of generic drug shortages as one reason why prices have seen such colossal increases.

Some of the solutions proposed in this *JAMA* editorial resemble Soviet-era attempts to regulate their economy that all proved disastrous. The *JAMA* authors make it appear impossible to predict competitive pressures in the generic drug arena. Their solution is for the federal government to enact new laws to protect generic manufacturers against the uncertainties of the marketplace, such as limiting the number of makers who could produce the same generic drug.

When I read this I thought, are educated people really this stupid? Every day in the private sector, projections are made for future inventory needs, often for products that have razor-thin margins. Yet when you walk into a grocery store, the shelves are consistently well-stocked, and shortages almost never occur. How do all these private-sector companies manage this without federal protection against overly optimistic projections?

Completely overlooked by the *JAMA* authors is the fact that when a free market is allowed to determine supply and demand, there are no shortages, and consumer prices usually go down over time (inflation-adjusted). There is no secret to making ample quantities of quality generic drugs. Yet consumers are being blatantly lied to as to why their costs for generic drugs are surging.

WE ARE MORE THAN A SUPPLEMENT SUPPLIER . . .

Much of Life Extension's® efforts go beyond making innovative dietary supplements. The reality is that our supporters help fund a variety of programs that challenge conventional dogma relating to human longevity and consumer justice. To reiterate what I said at the beginning of this chapter, no one has fought longer or harder against extortionist drug prices than Life Extension®. We have battled pharmaceutical interests for decades and won concessions in Congress and the courts that no one would have ever believed possible.

You're finally seeing news media revelations about the price gouging we predicted would inevitably happen back in the 1980s. The sad fact is that none of our politicians have the basic knowledge needed to rein in today's runaway healthcare costs. We at Life Extension®, on the other hand, have a 36-year track record of involvement in all ends of the pharmaceutical arena. We know the only impediment to slashing generic drug costs is citizen apathy that allows the FDA to continue enforcing a defacto monopoly that benefits the entrenched pharmaceutical establishment.

To enlist as an activist to combat high drug prices log on to: LifeExtension.com/consumer.

References

1. Available at: http://www.lifeextension.com/Magazine/2014/4/ Unsustainable-Cancer-Drug-Prices/Page-01. Accessed November 30, 2015.

2. Available at: http://www.lifeextension.com/Magazine/2014/9/ How-To-Turn-8-Pennies-Into-$600/Page-01. Accessed November 30, 2015.

3. Available at: http://www.lifeextension.com/Magazine/2012/4/ Lethal-Shortages/Page-01. Accessed November 30, 2015.

4. Available at: http://www.lifeextension.com/Magazine/2011/3/ No-Real-Healthcare-Cost-Crisis/Page-01. Accessed November 30, 2015.

5. Available at: http://www.lifeextension.com/Magazine/2009/9/ Why-American-Healthcare-is-Headed-for-Collapse/Page-01. Accessed November 30, 2015.

6. Available at: http://www.lifeextension.com/Magazine/2009/8/ The-Generic-Drug-Rip-Off/Page-02. Accessed November 30, 2015.

7. Available at: http://www.lifeextension.com/Magazine/2009/3/ FDA-Ending-the-Atrocities/Page-01. Accessed November 30, 2015.

8. Availableat:http://www.lifeextension.com/Magazine/2007/8/awsi/Page-01. Accessed November 30, 2015.

9. Availableat:http://www.lifeextension.com/Magazine/2007/4/awsi/Page-01. Accessed November 30, 2015.

10. Availableat:http://www.lifeextension.com/Magazine/2005/3/awsi/Page-01. Accessed November 30, 2015.

11. Availableat:http://www.lifeextension.com/Magazine/2004/4/awsi/Page-01. Accessed November 30, 2015.

12. Available at: http://www.lifeextension.com/Magazine/2002/10/awsi/Page-01. Accessed November 30, 2015.

13. Availableat:http://www.lifeextension.com/Magazine/2002/4/awsi/Page-01. Accessed November 30, 2015.

14. Availableat:http://www.lifeextension.com/Magazine/2000/2/awsi/Page-01. Accessed November 30, 2015.

15. Availableat:http://www.lifeextension.com/Magazine/2000/7/cover_story/Page-01. Accessed November 30, 2015.

16. Availableat:http://www.lifeextension.com/Magazine/2000/8/awsi/Page-01. Accessed November 30, 2015.

17. Availableat:http://www.lifeextension.com/Magazine/2000/9/awsi/Page-01. Accessed November 30, 2015.

18. Availableat:http://www.lifeextension.com/Magazine/2000/7/cover_story/Page-02. Accessed November 30, 2015.

19. Available at: http://www.lifeextension.com/Magazine/1999/6/awsi/Page-01. Accessed November 30, 2015.

20. Available at: http://www.lifeextension.com/Magazine/1998/12/awsi/Page-01. Accessed November 30, 2015.

21. Alpern JD, Stauffer WM, Kesselheim AS. High-cost generic drugs—implications for patients and policymakers. *N Engl J Med.* 2014;371(20):1859–62.

22. Available at: http://www.cbsnews.com/news/generic-drug-prices-skyrocketing/. Accessed November 30, 2015.

23. Available at: http://www.cbsnews.com/news/obamacare-60-minutes/. Accessed November 30, 2015.

24. Available at: http://www.lifeextension.com/about/lef-scientific-achievements-in-health-and-longevity_01. Accessed November 30, 2015.

"Unsustainable" Cancer Drug Prices

O VER 100 ONCOLOGISTS are protesting the outlandish prices charged for cancer drugs and how these inflated costs are economically "unsustainable."[1] Their exposé was published in a prestigious medical journal and received headline news coverage last year.[1,2] The more than 100 oncologists who authored this report noted that of twelve cancer drugs approved in 2012, eleven were priced above $100,000 per year.[1] Before relating the details, I ask readers to fathom who can afford $100,000 a year for one drug? This does not include hospital costs, physician fees, or other medications cancer patients typically require. Private insurance premiums are soaring in response to skyrocketing medical costs, along with governmental meddling. Federal healthcare programs face insolvency even without this kind of price gouging.

The oncologists protesting these high prices are experts in chronic myeloid leukemia, a bone marrow cancer that is responding unusually well to new cancer drugs. The dilemma these doctors disclose is that patients are surviving longer than expected . . . in some cases indefinitely . . . as long as they continue to receive their expensive drugs.[1,3] These doctors conclude that the prices of these drugs "are too high, unsustainable, may compromise access of needy patients to highly effective therapy, and are harmful to the sustainability of our national healthcare systems."[1] These revelations from inside the cancer establishment will not surprise Life Extension's followers, who long ago learned how regulatory strangleholds over drug development inflict harsh economic pain. Chronic Myelogenous Leukemia (also known as Chronic Myeloid Leukemia or CML) is a cancer of the blood and bone marrow.[4] It's one of four main kinds of leukemia. It is characterized by the increased and unregulated growth of predominantly myeloid cells in the bone marrow and the accumulation of these cells in the blood.[4] Treatment enhancements have been significant for this type of leukemia. In the 1960s, five-year overall survival rates were only 3–5%.[5] Five-year survival rates today are over 90% in those with chronic phase disease.[5,6] CML is one of the few cancers where meaningful treatment progress has occurred.[6]

COST PER MONTH OF ADDED LIFE

The more than 100 oncologists protesting the high prices are impressed with the anti-leukemic properties of these drugs. They note how some patients appear able to survive with chronic myeloid leukemia indefinitely . . . as long as they have access to the expensive medication(s).[1] The concern they raise is how individuals and/or society can ever afford the high prices, and why pharmaceutical companies need to charge so much after they earn back the costs of development.

Unlike patients with metastasized solid tumors (colon, lung, pancreatic), patients with chronic myeloid leukemia (CML) now live close to normal life spans, as long as they receive the appropriate drugs and adhere to treatment. In these patients, their CML condition has become different from cancers that sadly kill many patients within a year or two. The CML form of leukemia is now more similar to chronic disorders like diabetes and hypertension, where daily therapy is required to produce the benefit of long-term survival.[1] The problem is that patients stricken with CML are becoming the "financial victims" of the treatment success, having to pay outlandishly high prices forever to stay alive.

HOW HIGH?

Three drugs approved by the FDA in 2012 to treat leukemia are priced at the following astronomical levels:[7]

Ponatinib	$138,000
Bosutinib	$118,000
Bosutinib	Over $100,000

Older anti-leukemia drugs like imatinib (Gleevec®) were initially priced at nearly $30,000 a year when released in 2001. By 2012, the pharmaceutical company making Gleevec® increased the price to $92,000 a year.[8]

The annual costs for these anti-leukemia drugs are beyond the financial abilities of private industry, government, and 99% of individuals in the United States. One reason why these drugs in particular are a problem is that each leukemia patient may need to use one or a combination of these medications for decades. The economic unreality of all this is why more than 100 oncologists grouped together to alert the world that the high prices for these cancer drugs are "unsustainable."[1]

DEVELOPMENT COSTS LONG AGO PAID FOR

Pharmaceutical companies pretend they need to charge high prices to justify their expensive development costs. The more than 100 oncologists carefully examined this argument and found it to be unjustified. Gleevec®, for instance, quickly covered its research and development costs with its $30,000/year initial annual price. As it was approved for other indications, total revenue soared and it became a financial windfall for its maker (Novartis). Despite pleas by patients and advocates to lower the price of Gleevec®, it sells for more than three times its original price.[1,8] Who can afford to pay $92,000 a year for one drug?

COLLUSIVE BEHAVIOR AND HIGH PRICES

The drugs working so well against CML are in a class known as "tyrosine-kinase inhibitors."[1] There are now five tyrosine-kinase inhibiting drugs approved to treat CML, yet all five have annual price ranges of $92,000 to $138,000 in the United States. This is twice the price compared to Europe, where government health programs bargain for lower drug prices.[1] As the more than 100 oncologists noted in their published report, the price in South Korea for these same tyrosine-kinase inhibitors ranges from $21,000 to $28,000.[1] That's perhaps because the Koreans developed their own tyrosine-kinase inhibitor that sells for an annual price of only $21,500, thus forcing pharmaceutical companies to lower their price sharply downward compared to the United States and even Europe.

The more than 100 oncologists who authored the published report protesting the high prices state:

> A new branch of economics, called game theory, details how collusive behavior can tacitly maintain high prices over extended periods of time,

despite competitive markets, thus representing a form of collective monopoly.[1]

We at Life Extension® have alleged for decades that drug companies function like cartels in stomping out competition while maintaining monopolistic-like pricing. They do this in many ways that are quite open, such as filing lawsuits to delay the introduction of lower cost generics, and/or filing petitions with the FDA asking the agency to disallow a competitor's lower cost and sometimes superior product.[9]

It is interesting to note that some of the cancer-protective effects of nutrients like curcumin have been partially attributed to its tyrosine-kinase inhibiting properties. While curcumin has not yet been proven to be as specific as the drugs described in this chapter, a search on PubMed using the terms "curcumin and leukemia" reveals multiple mechanisms by which low-cost curcumin may prevent and treat a wide range of cancers.[10]

WHAT DO DRUGS REALLY COST TO DEVELOP?

There is a debate as to how much it really "costs" a pharmaceutical company to bring a new cancer drug to market. The sum of $2.6 billion[37] is often cited, though some independent experts put it as low as $60–90 million.[38] Whatever the real number, be assured it includes costs of development of the new drug that won FDA approval, all other drugs that failed, and ancillary expenses such as the cost of conducting the clinical trials, bonuses, salaries, infrastructures, royalties, advertising, and all kinds of perks to the doctors who prescribe the drugs.

As to how much a new drug really costs to develop, once a company sells about a billion dollars of a medication, most of the rest is profit. It's incredulous to claim that new cancer drugs are priced over $100,000 a year because they cost so much to develop. As you'll read later, much of the initial discovery costs are funded by non-profit entities involved in basic research. After the first two years of a successful drug launch, the "costs" of development are usually more than paid back.

HOW DRUG COMPANIES FLEECE THE PUBLIC

Before the federal government started picking up the tab for cancer drugs, there was at least an affordability factor that constrained how much pharmaceutical companies could charge. This changed in response to intensive lobbying by pharmaceutical interests that enabled passage of laws such as the Medicare Modernization Act of 2003. This Act resulted in the federal government paying full retail price for cancer drugs and prohibited the federal government from negotiating a lower price.[39] Even before the Medicare Modernization Act, the federal government was paying retail prices for cancer drugs under existing Medicare and Medicaid programs. Passage of the Affordable Care Act of 2010 enabled pharmaceutical companies to gouge virtually the entire American market with their outlandish prices.[40]

Consumers pay for these inflated drug prices in the form of higher private insurance premiums, higher deductibles, higher co-pays, and higher taxes. Medicare's date with insolvency will be hastened as it pays out tens of billions of excess dollars into pharmaceutical company coffers. Those who have employer-funded health insurance are paying a greater portion of their medical insurance premium, while healthcare inflation remains a major factor behind corporate and municipal bankruptcies.

I don't view it as a coincidence that since the passage of the Medicare Modernization Act, cancer drugs the federal government pays for (like Gleevec®) have spiraled upwards in price. This Act was written and enacted into law under intensive pressure from pharmaceutical lobbyists. We at Life Extension® vehemently opposed the Medicare Modernization Act that enabled pharmaceutical companies to charge full retail price for drugs paid for by federal tax/debt dollars. The obscene profits earned by a relatively small number of pharmaceutical companies provide them with virtually unlimited resources to influence Congress, the FDA, academia, the media, medical journals, and prescribing physicians in ways that go against the welfare of the American public.

HOW GLEEVEC® WAS DISCOVERED

Gleevec® was approved by the FDA in 2001, but the history of its discovery dates back to 1960, when scientists from the University of Pennsylvania School of Medicine and Institute for Cancer Research identified a genetic mutation in patients with CML (chronic myeloid leukemia).[48] The discovery meant that for the first time ever, scientists had discovered a genetic abnormality linked to a specific kind of cancer. This finding set off an explosion of research into the genetic causes of cancer. The next significant advance took place 13 years later through the work of researchers at the University of Chicago who found that the missing section of DNA that characterized CML had shifted to another chromosome, a phenomenon known as "trans-location."[49]

In the 1980s, researchers from the National Cancer Institute and Erasmus University identified the principal chromosomal cause of CML.[50] Later, in 1990, researchers at UCLA found this defective chromosome produced a protein that enhances tyrosine kinase activity, which changes the cell's normal genetic instructions and enables aberrant cell growth and division.[50]

With the discovery that a single enzyme could cause the development of CML, researchers were given a rare opportunity. The genetic target was clear, and the development of a drug that could inhibit the protein that enhanced tyrosine kinase could proceed rationally. Work began in the early 1990s on the discovery of tyrosine kinase inhibitors by researchers at Novartis, who collaborated with scientists from the Howard Hughes Medical Institute and other research centers.[50-53]

The first Phase I study began in 1998.[53,54] The results of these preliminary studies showed that over 98% of CML patients who took the drug were responding.[54] Most patients experienced a significant reduction in the number of white blood cells and a reduction or disappearance in the number of cells containing the cancer-triggering chromosome. Word of the drug's effectiveness spread rapidly in the CML community, and tremendous pressure was applied for Novartis to make more Gleevec® available so more patients could participate in the clinical trials. As more Gleevec® was made available, thousands of CML patients had their death sentence lifted. The FDA approved Gleevec® in 2001, ten weeks after Novartis submitted the application.[55]

This brief historical description shows how drug discovery is often initiated by non-profit research centers and then much later brought to fruition by commercial pharmaceutical companies. Some of the scientists involved in the early development of Gleevec® are part of the more than 100 oncologists who authored the report that seeks to lower the price of these tyrosine kinase inhibiting cancer drugs (such as Gleevec®). While commercial companies play a vital role in drug development, it is so often research funded by non-profit entities that identifies a breakthrough "target" for which to develop a drug.

NOVARTIS ACCUSED OF PAYING ILLEGAL KICKBACKS TO DOCTORS

Two of the five overpriced anti-leukemic drugs identified by oncologists are Gleevec® (imatinib) and Tasigna® (nilotinib), both made by Swiss pharmaceutical behemoth Novartis.[41] US prosecutors have brought civil-fraud charges against Novartis for allegedly paying kickbacks to physicians to prescribe their diabetes and anti-hypertension drugs.[42] Novartis claims the money was paid to doctors to speak at education programs around the United States. The charges against Novartis allege speaking fees, lavish dinners, and vacations illegally provided to doctors totaling nearly $65 million.[42] This money of course is all included in the "cost" of drug development.

HOW MUCH THE DOCTORS WERE PAID

The lawsuit against Novartis alleges that the doctors (speakers) were usually paid $750–$1,500 per program, with some earning as much as $3,000 to talk at fancy restaurants, or in one case, on a fishing boat in Florida.[42] The government's lawsuit further alleges that one doctor was paid $3,750 for speaking to the same four doctors about a Novartis drug five times in a nine-month period.[43] In another allegation, a doctor was paid $500 to speak at an expensive Manhattan restaurant dinner attended by his friends. Many of these so-called "speaking engagements" occurred with less than three doctors attending, or in some cases, no doctor attending, in which case I suppose, Novartis paid the doctor to speak to himself at a fancy dinner paid for by Novartis.

The government's lawsuit describes dinners where the price per person attending ranged from $672 to over $1,000.[42] I feel somewhat out of place here, but I have never been to a dinner where each guest ran up a tab like this for food and beverages. The lawsuit alleges that few slides were ever shown at these speaking engagements. "Instead, Novartis simply wined and dined the doctors at high-end restaurants with astronomical costs."[43] Not all the restaurants where Novartis paid doctors to speak and covered the meals were high-end. Some were sports bars (such as Hooters) with so many blaring TV screens (and no private room) that it would have been impossible to make a scientific presentation.[42]

NOT THE FIRST TIME FOR NOVARTIS

This is not the first time Novartis has been accused of paying doctors kickbacks to prescribe drugs that are often overpriced compared to generics, and therefore defraud government programs like Medicare and Medicaid.[44,45] In 2010, the same unit of Novartis pled guilty to misdemeanor violations and paid $422.5 million to settle civil and criminal charges that it illegally marketed certain pharmaceutical products and paid doctors kickbacks to prescribe it.[44] Novartis denies the charges that it illegally paid kickbacks to doctors in the current civil-fraud lawsuit.[45]

OUTLANDISH COST OF CANCER DRUGS

Pharmaceutical companies know that Medicare, Medicaid, and many insurance companies pay unlimited amounts of money for their drugs. What few consumers realize is that they are bearing the cost of these over-priced drugs in the form of higher insurance premiums, higher deductibles, higher co-pays, more exclusions, higher taxes, and higher interest costs on the national debt as government programs pay these outlandish prices. Pharmaceutical companies price gouge the public by charging the *obscene prices* you see on the following two pages:

Brand Name	Generic Name	Type of Cancer	Cost of Drugs
Avastin®	*(bevacizumab)*	Breast Cancer Colon	$100,000[11], $55,000 (2004)[12], $85,000 (2011)[13]
Avastin ®	*(bevacizumab)*	Brain Cancer that recurred	$43,000[14]
Iclusig®	*(ponatinib)*	Chronic Myeloid Leukemia (CML)	$138,000[15]
Bosulif®	*(bosutinib)*	Chronic Myeloid Leukemia (CML)	$118,000[15]
Gleevec®	*(imatinib)*	Chronic Myeloid Leukemia (CML)	$30,000 (2001) $92,000 (2012)[15]
Erbitux®	*(cetuximab)*	Colon Cancer, Lung Cancer	$80,000[16]
Cometriq®	*(cabozantinib)*	Thyroid Cancer	$99,000[17]
Erivedge®	*(vismodegib*®*)*	Skin Cancer	$75,000[18]
Herceptin®	*(trastuzumab)*	Breast Cancer	$70,000[19]
Camptosar®	*(irinotecan)*	Stage IV Colon Cancer	$44,087[20]
Eloxatin®	*(oxaliplatin)*	Stage IV Colon Cancer	$60,179[20]
Synribo®	*(omacetaxine)*	Chronic Myeloid Leukemia (CML)	$28,000 for induction and $14,000 for a maintenance course[15]
Kadcyla®	*(ado-trastuzumabemtansine)*	Breast Cancer	$94,000[21]
Nexavar®	*(sorafenib)*	Liver Cancer Kidney Cancer	$80,000[22] $96,000[22]
Perjeta®	*(pertuzumab)*	Breast Cancer	$106,200[23] (based on 18-month course of treatment)
Provenge®	*(sipuleucel-T)*	Prostate Cancer	$93,000[24]
Proleukin®	*(aldesleukin)*	Kidney Cancer, Metastatic Melanoma	Up to $3,925 per dose, $109,900 per course based on 28 doses, $549,500 per year based on 5 courses[25,26]

Brand Name	Generic Name	Type of Cancer	Cost of Drugs
Sutent®	(sunitinib malate)	Kidney, pancreatic and GI Cancer	$48,720[27]
Tarceva®	(erlotinib)	Non-Small Cell Lung Cancer $31,00028	$31,000[28]
Xalkori®	(crizotinib)	Non-Small Cell Lung Cancer	$115,000[29]
Xgeva®	(denosumab)	Metastasis to Bones	$6,600[30]
Xtandi®	(enzalutamide)	prostate Cancer (metastatic castration-resistant-mCrpC)	$59,600[31]
Votrient®	(pazopanib)	Kidney Cancer Sarcomas[33] (2012)	$93,000[32] (based on 800 mg per day)
Yervoy®	(ipilimumab)	Melanoma	about $116,000[34] (about $29,000 per infusion, 4 needed)
Zelboraf®	(vemurafenib)	Metastatic Melanoma	$112,800[35] (2012) $60,000[29] (2011)
Zytiga®	(abiraterone)	Prostate Cancer (castration-resistant-CrpC)	$60,000[36]

A BROKEN SYSTEM!

The magnitude of pharmaceutical company malfeasance is incomprehensible to the lay public. Consumers know healthcare costs are rising, yet cures for most killer diseases remain elusive. New cancer drugs that add only a few agonizing months of survival are laden with such severe side effects that many patients reject them altogether. Some cancer patients say no to these over-priced drugs to spare their families insolvency. Pharmaceutical companies today seek to gain FDA approval of patented drugs that may temporarily shrink tumor volume, but don't always meaningfully improve patient survival. The leukemia drugs described in this chapter are the exception when it comes to long-term efficacy and relative safety.[5,6]

Richard Nixon declared war on cancer in 1971.[46] Hundreds of billions of dollars of federal funds have been spent on research. Cancer patients survive longer today, but missing are the miracle cures envisioned 43 years ago. Long-term side effects from radiation or chemotherapy cause deaths from stroke, heart failure, or immune impairment. These cancer therapy-induced deaths are not "counted" in the cancer statistics, thus enabling the cancer establishment to pretend they are making more progress than they really are.[47]

OUR "DIFFERENT" APPROACH TO CANCER TREATMENT

We at *Life Extension®* fund clinical cancer research aimed at discovering if protocols that involve dozens of drugs, nutrients, and other therapies can produce long-term complete responses, i.e. cures. We have spent millions of dollars testing a wide array of "other" companies' therapies in unique combinations to see if we can attain remissions or complete responses. Our clinical successes in some cases are unprecedented, yet we don't own the intellectual property (i.e. the drugs) that enables these successes to occur. Instead, we publish the results of our research in books like *Disease Prevention and Treatment*, on our website, or disseminate to our members through our health advisory staff.

We never use placebos in cancer patients as we believe this to be genocide. All cancer patients who enter our clinical trials receive therapies that are intended to cure (or mitigate) their underlying malignancy. Life Extension® does not believe any human being should be treated as an experimental lab animal. Support of our cancer research initiatives is made possible through our supporters' contributions and supplement purchases.

References

1. Experts in Chronic Myeloid Leukemia. The price of drugs for chronic myeloid leukemia (CML) is a reflection of the unsustainable prices of cancer drugs: from the perspective of a large group of CML experts. *Blood.* 2013 May 30;121(22):4439–42.
2. Available at: http://money.cnn.com/2013/04/25/news/economy/cancer-drug-cost/. Accessed May 21, 2013.
3. Gambacorti-Passerini C, Antolini L, Mahon FX, et al. Multicenter independent assessment of outcomes in chronic myeloid leukemia patients treated with imatinib. *J Natl Cancer Inst.* 2011 Apr 6;103(7):553–61.
4. Available at: http://www.cancer.org/cancer/leukemia-chronicmyeloidcml/detailedguide/leukemia-chronic-myeloid-myelogenous-what-is-c-m-l. Accessed June 17, 2013.
5. Available at: http://www.medicalnewstoday.com/articles/252113.php. Accessed May 21, 2013.
6. Available at: http://www.medicalnewstoday.com/releases/240653.php. Accessed May 21, 2013.
7. Available at: http://www.genengnews.com/gen-articles/cancer-s-bitter-medicine/4913/. Accessed June 17, 2013.
8. Available at: http://www.pslweb.org/liberationnews/news/oncologists-protest-cancer-drugs-cost.html. Accessed June 17, 2013.
9. Available at: http://www.ftc.gov/os/2011/08/2011genericdrugreport.pdf. Accessed May 21, 2013.
10. Available at: http://cdn.elsevier.com/assets/pdf_file/0006/115719/current-problems-in-cancer-article-1.pdf. Accessed May 21, 2013.
11. Available at: http://www.news-medical.net/health/Avastin-(Bevacizumab)-Price.aspx. Accessed June 19, 2013.

12. Available at: http://www.bankrate.com/finance/insurance/insuring-costs-cancer-1.aspx. Accessed June 7, 2013.

13. Available at: http://www.drugs.com/newdrugs/fda-approves-avastin-combination-chemotherapy-first-line-most-common-type-lung-cancer-1140.html. Accessed June 18, 2013.

14. Available at: http://news.yahoo.com/avastin-fails-studies-brain-tumor-patients-133937951.html. Accessed June 7, 2013.

15. Available at: http://www.medscape.com/viewarticle/803415. Accessed June 7, 2013.

16. Available at: http://www.bloomberg.com/apps/news?pid=n ewsarchive&sid=a477Nm93JYxM. Accessed June 7, 2013.

17. Available at: http://seekingalpha.com/article/1487722-exelixis-and-cabozantinib-asco-2013-highlights. Accessed June 7, 2013.

18. Available at: http://prescriptions.blogs.nytimes.com/2012/01/30/f-d-a-approves-drug-for-an-advanced-skin-cancer/. Accessed June 7, 2013.

19. Available at: http://www.medicalnewstoday.com/articles/250912.php. Accessed June 19, 2013.

20. Mullins CD, Hsiao FY, Onukwugha E, Pandya NB, Hanna N. Comparative and cost-effectiveness of oxaliplatin-based or irinotecan-based regimens compared with 5-fluorouracil/leucovorin alone among US elderly stage IV colon cancer patients. *Cancer.* 2012 Jun 15;118(12):3173–81.

21. Available at: http://www.nytimes.com/2013/02/23/business/fda-approves-breast-cancer-drug.html?_r=0. Accessed June 7, 2013.

22. Available at: http://www.forbes.com/sites/matthewherper/2012/03/19/how-to-charge-1-6-million-for-a-new-drug-and-get-away-with-it/. Accessed June 7, 2013.

23. Available at: http://www.nytimes.com/2012/06/09/business/genentech-wins-approval-for-new-breast-cancer-drug.html?_r=0. Accessed June 7, 2013.

24. Available at: http://seekingalpha.com/article/1413381-bracing-for-dendreon-q1-2013-earnings-all-eyes-on-provenge. Accessed June 7, 2013.

25. Available at: http://dailymed.nlm.nih.gov/dailymed/lookup.cfm?setid=a588140c-f9ed-4a9b-a9a6-bf3daafd8a5a. Accessed January 21, 2014.

26. Available at: http://www.goodrx.com/proleukin/what-is. Accessed January 21, 2014.

27. Available at: http://www.bloomberg.com/apps/news?pid=newsarchive&sid=aER.9zj2HmSk. Accessed June 7, 2013.

28. Available at: http://www.nytimes.com/2005/07/12/business/worldbusiness/12iht-drugs.html?_r=0. Accessed June 7, 2013.

29. Available at: http://www.forbes.com/sites/matthewherper/2011/08/26/pfizer-wins-approval-for-xalkori-lung-cancer-drug-that-heralds-age-of-expensive-personalized-medicines/. Accessed June 7, 2013.

30. Available at: http://prescriptions.blogs.nytimes.com/2010/11/18/f-d-a-approves-a-bone-drug-for-cancer-patients/. Accessed June 7, 2013.

31. Available at: http://www.nytimes.com/2012/09/01/business/fda-approves-prostate-cancer-drug.html. Accessed June 7, 2013.

32. Available at: http://cashcard.lc.healthtrans.com/Pages/PharmacyLocator.aspx?host=default. Accessed June 7, 2013.

33. Available at: http://www.fda.gov/NewsEvents/Newsroom/PressAnnouncements/ucm302065.htm. Accessed June 7, 2013.

34. Available at: http://www.pharmacytimes.com/publications/health-system-edition/2012/November2012/Formulary-Drug-Review-Ipilimumab-Yervoy. Accessed June 7, 2013.

35. Available at: http://www.webmd.com/melanoma-skin-cancer/news/20120222/zelboraf-may-double-survival-for-some-melanoma-patients. Accessed June 7, 2013.

36. Available at: http://www.nytimes.com/2011/06/28/health/28prostate.html. Accessed June 7, 2013.

37. Mullard, Asher. "New drugs cost US $2.6 billion to develop." *Nature Reviews Drug Discovery.* 13, no. 12 (2014):877.

38. Light D, Lexchin J. Pharmaceutical research and development: what do we get for all that money? *BJM.* 2012 344:4348.

39. Available at: http://www.gpo.gov/fdsys/pkg/PLAW-108publ173/html/PLAW-108publ173.htm. Accessed May 21, 2013.

40. Available at: http://www.gpo.gov/fdsys/pkg/PLAW-111publ148/html/PLAW-111publ148.htm. Accessed May 21, 2013.

41. Available at: http://www.bloomberg.com/news/2012-10-25/novartis-cannibalizes-gleevec-to-boost-new-cancer-drug.html. Accessed January 21, 2014.

42. Available at: http://online.wsj.com/news/articles/SB10001424127887324474004578447053898340538. Accessed January 27, 2014.

43. Available at: http://www.tampabay.com/news/courts/lawsuit-pharmaceutical-company-gave-kickbacks-to-florida-doctors/2119133. Accessed January 21, 2014.

44. Available at: http://www.justice.gov/opa/pr/2010/September/10-civ-1102.html. Accessed January 22, 2014.

45. Available at: http://www.reuters.com/article/2013/04/23/us-novartis-fraud-lawsuit-idUSBRE93M1C920130423. Accessed January 22, 2014.

46. Available at: http://dtp.nci.nih.gov/timeline/noflash/milestones/m4_nixon.htm. Accessed January 22, 2014.

47. Available at: http://www.cancer.net/survivorship/long-term-side-effects-cancer-treatment. Accessed January 22, 2014.

48. Nowell PC, Hungerford DA. A minute chromosome in human chronic granulocytic leukaemia. *Science.* 1960 132:164–172.

49. Rowley D. A new consistent chromosomal abnormality in chronic myelogenous leukaemia identified by quinacrine fluorescence and Giemsa staining. *Nature.* 1973 243:290–293.

50. Available at: http://asheducationbook.hematologylibrary. org/content/2008/1/418.full. Accessed January 22, 2014.

51. Available at: http://www.hhmi.org/news/five-year-study-shows-gleevecs-potency-against-chronic-myeloid-leukemia. Accessed January 22, 2014.

52. Druker BJ, Tamura S, Buchdunger E, et al. Effects of a selective inhibitor of the Abl tyrosine kinase on the growth of Bcr-Abl positive cells. *Nat Med.* 1996 May;2(5):561–6.

53. Available at: http://www.cancer.gov/researchandfunding/ extramural/cancercenters/accomplishments/gleevec. Accessed May 21, 2013.

54. Available at: http://bloodjournal.hematologylibrary.org/ content/105/7/2640.full. Accessed May 21, 2013.

55. Available at: http://www.innovation.org/index.cfm/ StoriesofInnovation/InnovatorStories/The_Story_of_ Gleevec. Accessed January 22, 2014.

Legal Murder

N O ONE KNOWS EXACTLY how many Americans were killed by Vioxx®. According to Dr. David Graham, the hero who defied his corrupt FDA superiors, Vioxx® caused 88,000 to 139,000 excess cases of heart attack and stroke.[1,2] This carnage occurred as Merck (the maker of Vioxx®) worked closely with high-level FDA officials to suppress data showing the lethal dangers of this once-popular arthritis drug.[3,4] According to a review published in the *Archives of Internal Medicine*, Merck held back initial data showing Vioxx® caused an increase in heart attack and stroke risk.[5] It took three more years of patients needlessly dying before Vioxx® was pulled off the market. The FDA never mandated Vioxx® be banned. As lawsuits started piling up, Merck made a business decision to withdraw Vioxx® worldwide, while denying there was a safety issue.[6]

MERCK PLEADS GUILTY TO CRIMINAL CHARGES

After a seven-year Justice Department investigation, Merck pled guilty to a criminal misdemeanor that it illegally promoted Vioxx® and deceived the government about the drug's safety.[7] Merck paid the federal government a $950 million fine. It has also paid over $4 billion in compensation to victims (or their family members) for the side effects Vioxx® caused, along with punitive damages for covering up the lethal dangers.[7] Before it was withdrawn, Merck racked up $11 billion in Vioxx® sales.[8] So with the criminal fine paid to the government and the money paid out so far to victims, Merck appears to be billions of dollars ahead financially by knowingly selling a drug that killed tens of thousands of human beings!

EGREGIOUS COVER-UP

Four years before Vioxx® was withdrawn, the results from a large clinical trial were published comparing patients using naproxen or Vioxx®. The findings showed a 500% increased risk of heart attack in Vioxx® users compared to those taking naproxen.[9] This trial was designed, performed, and paid for by the drug industry. The findings from this trial should have resulted in the FDA withdrawing approval of Vioxx®. Instead, the drug industry (working in cahoots with the FDA) came up with a ridiculous upside-down analysis of the data. They concluded that Vioxx® did not cause a 500% increase in heart attacks, but instead that naproxen resulted in a 500% decrease in heart attack incidence.[10]

Dr. David Graham is the senior epidemiologist in the FDA's Office of Drug Safety. Dr. Graham knew that naproxen did not reduce heart attack risk by 500%. When Dr. Graham saw how data from this study was being manipulated to cover up Vioxx's lethal dangers, he broke rank with corrupt FDA officials. Dr. Graham's battle to expose the lethal dangers of Vioxx® almost got him fired from the FDA.

GOVERNMENT DOESN'T CARE ABOUT VICTIMS

As most of you know, the intentional killing of a human is a felony, often punishable by life in prison (or worse). In the Justice Department's settlement with Merck, there is no discussion of murder. Instead, Merck agreed to plead guilty to FDA "regulatory" violations involving its promotion of Vioxx® to rheumatoid arthritis patients when it was approved only to treat osteoarthritis. Merck also pled guilty to misleading Medicaid officials about the safety of Vioxx®.[11] Dr. David Graham estimates that Vioxx® directly killed more Americans than died during the entire Vietnam War.[9] Yet nowhere in the criminal settlement agreement does Merck have to admit to "intentionally killing people."

It appears that the Justice Department is not concerned by the human body count. The settlement only requires that Merck admit they failed to comply with FDA and Medicaid regulations.[12] Interestingly, there are published studies showing that Vioxx® was effective against rheumatoid arthritis, but such data is irrelevant since the FDA had not "approved" Vioxx® for this indication.[11] Our government was more concerned about "regulatory violations" than accurately assessing scientific facts about Vioxx® in the treatment of rheumatoid arthritis. The rationale you'll read next for Merck not being charged with felony murder demonstrates the insidious influence pharmaceutical behemoths exert over the federal government.[13]

WHY PHARMACEUTICAL COMPANIES AREN'T CRIMINALLY PROSECUTED

Medicare and Medicaid pay out such a large portion of this nation's healthcare costs that pharmaceutical companies must maintain access to these government spigots to remain in business. If a drug company is convicted of "serious healthcare fraud," they are automatically excluded from receiving federal payouts. To protect the financial interests of large pharmaceutical companies, the federal government works out specials deals that enable them to avoid accountability for their illicit actions. In recent years, our government has allowed pharmaceutical companies to escape felony fraud charges, or allows a shell company-subsidiary to take the blame for the parent company's misdeeds. This is analogous to you committing a murder, but persuading a terminal cancer patient to take the blame for it, and prosecutors then letting you off the hook.

Vioxx® is in a class of drugs known as COX-II inhibitors. Another drug in this class approved by the FDA was Bextra® made by pharmaceutical behemoth Pfizer. Bextra® was also withdrawn because of increased risks of heart attacks, strokes, and deaths in patients prescribed it.[14–16] As we reported in 2010, Pfizer was allowed to use a subsidiary shell company to plead guilty to a criminal charge that it fraudulently sold Bextra®.[17] The fraud was based on Pfizer promoting Bextra®'s use in higher doses to relieve acute surgical pain, something the drug was never approved for.[18] Using a subsidiary to plead guilty to the Bextra® charges enabled Pfizer to continue receiving lucrative Medicare/Medicaid reimbursement on its other drugs. By allowing the Vioxx® atrocities to be settled on misdemeanor charges instead of felony counts, Merck will continue receiving billions of dollars of annual payments from Medicare/Medicaid.

BEXTRA®'S FATAL SIDE EFFECTS OVERLOOKED BY FDA

In an analysis presented at the American Heart Association, Bextra® was shown to more than double the risk of heart attack or stroke. The lead author of this study commented that, "This is a time bomb waiting to go off."[19]

Pfizer paid a settlement to the federal government of $1.195 billion for the fraudulent marketing of Bextra®.[20] The record financial payout was not because Bextra® injured and killed arthritis patients. The fine was to settle government claims that Pfizer illegally promoted the sale of Bextra® for uses and dosages that the FDA specifically declined to approve. Just as with Vioxx®, the government bases its Bextra® fine on regulatory violations instead of the fact that human beings were killed!

NO EQUAL JUSTICE

The slap-on-the-wrist settlements of the Vioxx® and Bextra® charges represent an egregious evasion of laws that are supposed to prohibit companies engaged in "serious healthcare fraud" from receiving tax dollars. Of course none of the individual perpetrators at drug companies that caused these horrific numbers of deaths ever have to worry about jail time.

If a supplement company owner knowingly sold a product that caused even one death, he would likely face decades in prison. As you'll read in another chapter of this book, a man named Jay Kimball sold a drug (liquid deprenyl) that harmed no one, but he was sentenced to 13 years in prison. The wrongful prosecution of Jay Kimball represents one of the worst miscarriages of justice in the history of the American jurisprudence. In comparing Jay Kimball's case to the real crimes of Merck and Pfizer, the FDA did not even attempt to show that Jay's liquid deprenyl harmed anyone. The FDA merely cited "regulatory violations" involving his improper export of his liquid deprenyl to other countries. The result was 12 years in jail for Jay Kimball and financial ruination for his family.[21]

Merck and Pfizer knowingly sold drugs (Vioxx® and Bextra®) that killed tens of thousands of Americans, yet they continue receiving billions of Medicare/Medicaid dollars each year, with no one facing jail time, while their executives lead lavish lifestyles.

COVERING UP OF VIOXX'S LETHAL DANGERS

By April 2001, Merck had compiled internal data from two large human trials showing a staggering three-fold increase in total mortality (deaths) in patients using Vioxx®.[22] In articles that reported the results of these trials, analyses and statistical tests of the mortality data were obscured. Even the study author's conclusion regarding safety of Vioxx® was absurdly stated as the drug being "well tolerated."[23]

Data submitted to the FDA was manipulated to understate the higher numbers of deaths in Vioxx® users. For example, if heart attack or stroke deaths occurred more than 14 days after Vioxx® was discontinued, it was often omitted. Just imagine how many heart attack and stroke victims stopped taking Vioxx® because arthritis was no longer their major medical concern. Paralyzed stroke patients, for instance, have little need for Vioxx®, yet many of these stroke victims die more than 14 days after discontinuing Vioxx®.

After the VIGOR study was published showing a 500% increase in myocardial infarction (heart attack) in Vioxx® users,[24] Merck directed its sales force to provide physicians with a distorted picture of the relevant scientific evidence. For instance, Merck sent a bulletin to its Vioxx® sales force of more than 3,000 representatives that ordered:

DO NOT INITIATE DISCUSSIONS ON THE FDA ARTHRITIS ADVISORY COMMITTEE . . . OR THE RESULTS OF THE . . . VIGOR STUDY.[25]

The Merck bulletin further advised that if a physician inquired about the VIGOR study, the sales representative should indicate that the study showed a gastrointestinal benefit and then say, "I cannot discuss the study with you."[25]

Merck further instructed its sales reps to show those doctors who asked whether Vioxx® caused myocardial infarction a pamphlet called "The Cardiovascular Card." This pamphlet, prepared by Merck's marketing department, indicated that Vioxx® was associated with 1/8 the mortality from cardiovascular causes of that found with other anti-inflammatory drugs. The Cardiovascular Card, however, provided a misleading picture of the evidence on Vioxx®. The card did not include any data from the VIGOR study that showed a 500% increase in heart attack risk. Instead, it presented a pooled analysis of preapproval studies, in most of which low doses of Vioxx® were used for a short time. None of these studies were designed to assess cardiovascular safety, and none included a proper determination of cardiovascular events. In fact, FDA experts had publicly expressed "serious concerns" to the FDA's advisory committee about using the preapproval studies as evidence of Vioxx's cardiovascular safety.

The cover-up of the lethal dangers of Vioxx® spanned a period of years, all the while tens of thousands of innocent victims worldwide perished needlessly. Merck continues to deny there is any safety problem with Vioxx®.

MERCK CONTROLS TIMING OF ANNOUNCEMENT OF GUILTY PLEA

Even for a company as huge as Merck, pleading guilty to criminal misdemeanors is embarrassing. While the credibility of pharmaceutical companies has sunk to an all-time low, they still pretend to care about the public's health. Merck's guilty plea was announced the day before Thanksgiving (2011), which is one of the busiest travel days of the year and a time when the fewest people are paying attention to the news. Talk about absolute power: Merck avoids felony charges, jail time for executives, and embarrassing publicity, all while keeping billions of surplus dollars on

Vioxx® sales. Jay Kimball, on the other hand, was incarcerated for 13 years and his family left indigent.

WE WARNED MEMBERS ABOUT DANGERS OF COX-2 INHIBITING DRUGS

While Merck was bombarding the public with television commercials claiming that one little pill a day of Vioxx® took away arthritis pain, Life Extension® warned its members about the lethal dangers of Vioxx® and other drugs that inhibit only the COX-2 enzyme. We knew that Vioxx's mechanism of action would result in sharply higher rates of coronary artery blockage and ischemic stroke. So did scientists who evaluated Vioxx® before the FDA approved it. Despite the criminal guilty plea, the $950 million settlement, and its withdrawal of Vioxx® worldwide, Merck still denies any wrongdoing on the part of its higher level executives or the company itself.

MORE GUILTY PLEAS BY BIG PHARMA

As we were finalizing our article, GlaxoSmithKline had reached the largest illegal drug settlement to date, agreeing to pay $3 billion and plead guilty to criminal charges that included the drugs Avandia® and Paxil®.[26] Avandia® is a drug used to treat type II diabetes. Vascular disease is the leading cause of mortality in diabetic patients.[27,28] In a study of 227,571 patients, those receiving Avandia® were 27% more likely to suffer strokes, 25% more likely to develop heart failure, and 14% more likely to die compared to those taking another anti-diabetic drug called Actos®.[29,30] Avandia® increased the very diseases that diabetic patients are most vulnerable to—and Glaxo covered up these deadly side effects![31]

Paxil® is a drug prescribed to treat depression. After years of cover-up, Glaxo sent a letter to physicians admitting that the risk of suicidal behavior was 6.7 times higher in study subjects taking Paxil® compared to placebo. Suicide risk is high in depressed individuals, yet Glaxo covered up suicidal risks as it promoted the so-called "benefits" of Paxil® in treating depression.[32] Glaxo's guilty plea to criminal charges was announced two days before July 4, 2012, another busy travel time when few Americans are reading the news.

Two weeks after Glaxo's record settlement, Johnson and Johnson agreed to pay $2.2 billion for its illegal marketing of the drug Risperdal® to demented elderly patients.[33] Risperdal® is approved mainly to treat schizophrenia, but is associated with a number of deadly side effects including high blood sugar, irregular pulse, and blood pressure irregularities.[34] The most troubling side effect of Risperdal® is impairment of judgment and thinking, which is the last thing a demented patient needs.[34]

In each of these cases, pharmaceutical companies were promoting drugs that worsened the diseases they were intending to treat. We don't yet know how their guilty pleas will be manipulated so they don't lose out on lucrative Medicare/Medicaid reimbursement.

References

1. Available at: http://www.consumersunion.org/pub/core_health_care/001651.html. Accessed April 12, 2012.

2. Available at: http://www.finance.senate.gov/imo/media/doc/111804dgtest.pdf. Accessed April 12, 2012.

3. Available at: http://www.marshall-attorneys.com/Press/2004_11_01_WSJ.htm. Accessed April 12, 2012.

4. Horton R. Vioxx, the implosion of Merck, and aftershocks at the FDA. *Lancet.* 2004 Dec 4–10;364(9450):1995–6.

5. Ross JS, Madigan D, Hill KP, Egilman DS, Wang Y, Krumholz HM. Pooled analysis of rofecoxib placebo-controlled clinical trial data: lessons for postmarket pharmaceutical safety surveillance. *Arch Intern Med.* 2009 Nov 23;169(21):1976–85.

6. Available at: http://hcrenewal.blogspot.com/2011/12/merck-admits-little-while-settling.html. Accessed January 18, 2012.

7. Available at: http://wprsam.com/news/articles/2011/nov/22/merck-to-pay-nearly-1-billion-to-settle-us-charges/. Accessed April 12, 2012.

8. Available at: http://www.examiner.com/health-in-los-angeles/vioxx-settlement-hits-merck-for-950-million. Accessed January 20, 2012.

9. Available at: http://www.naturalnews.com/011401.html. Accessed January 25, 2012.

10. Available at: http://fl1.findlaw.com/news.findlaw.com/hdocs/docs/vioxx/111804singh.pdf. Accessed February 25, 2012.

11. Available at: http://www.businessweek.com/news/2011-12-05/merck-to-plead-guilty-pay-950-million-in-u-s-vioxx-probe.html. Accessed January 27, 2012.

12. Available at: http://www.bloomberg.com/news/2011-11-22/merck-agrees-to-pay-950-million-to-settle-u-s-government-s-vioxx-probe.html. Accessed February 8, 2012.

13. Available at: http://www.medscape.com/viewarticle/538025. Accessed February 15, 2012.

14. Available at: http://www.medicinenet.com/script/main/art.asp?articlekey=46601. Accessed February 15, 2012.

15. Roumie CL, Mitchel EF Jr, Kaltenbach L, Arbogast PG, Gideon P, Griffin MR. Nonaspirin NSAIDs, cyclooxygenase 2 inhibitors, and the risk for stroke. *Stroke*. 2008 Jul;39(7):2037–45.

16. Roumie CL, Choma NN, Kaltenbach L, Mitchel EF Jr, Arbogast PG, Griffin MR. Non-aspirin NSAIDs, cyclooxygenase-2 inhibitors and risk for cardiovascular events-stroke, acute myocardial infarction, and death from coronary heart disease. *Pharmacoepidemiol Drug Saf*. 2009 Nov;18(11):1053–63.

17. Available at http://www.lef.org/magazine/mag2011/jun2011_Obscene-Profits-Over-Human-Life_01.htm. Accessed March 8, 2012.

18. Available at: http://www.doj.state.wi.us/absolutenm/
templates/template_share.aspx?articleid=837&zoneid=4.
Accessed April 12, 2012.

19. Available at: http://www.medscape.com/viewarticle/538008.
Accessed February 22, 2012.

20. Available at: http://www.hhs.gov/news/
press/2009pres/09/20090902a.html. Accessed February
22, 2012.

21. Available at: http://www.proliberty.com/observer/20001201.
htm. Accessed April 12, 2012.

22. Available at: http://www.cbsnews.com/stories/2008/04/15/
health/webmd/main4018030.shtml. Accessed February 23,
2012.

23. Available at: http://www.bloomberg.com/apps/news?
pid=newsarchive&sid=a5z.VogSbbXo&refer=home.
Accessed February 24, 2012.

24. Bombardier C, Laine L, Reicin A, et al. VIGOR Study Group.
Comparison of upper gastrointestinal toxicity of rofecoxib
and naproxen in patients with rheumatoid arthritis. VIGOR
Study Group. *N Engl J Med*. 2000 Nov 23;343(21):1520–8, 2
p following 1528.

25. Available at: http://www.nejm.org/doi/full/10.1056/
NEJMp058136. Accessed February 24, 2012.

26. Available at: http://www.nytimes.com/2012/07/03/business/
glaxosmithkline-agrees-to-pay-3-billion-in-fraud-settlement.
html?_r=1&pagewanted=all. Accessed July 25, 2012.

27. Available at: http://www.world-heart-federation.org/
cardiovascular-health/cardiovascular-disease-risk-factors/
diabetes/. Accessed July 25, 2012.

28. Haffner SM, Lehto S, Rönnemaa T, Pyörälä K, Laakso M. Mortality from coronary heart disease in subjects with type 2 diabetes and in nondiabetic subjects with and without prior myocardial infarction. *N Engl J Med*. 1998 Jul 23;339(4):229–34.

29. Available at: http://www.cbsnews.com/2100-204_162-6627074.html. Accessed July 25, 2012.

30. Graham DJ, Ouellet-Hellstrom R, MaCurdy TE, et al. Risk of acute myocardial infarction, stroke, heart failure, and death in elderly Medicare patients treated with rosiglitazone or pioglitazone. *JAMA.* 2010 Jul 28;304(4):411–8.

31. Available at: http://www.drugwatch.com/2012/07/03/glaxosmithkline-pays-3-billion-for-illegal-drug-marketing/. Accessed July 25, 2012.

32. Available at: http://us.gsk.com/docs-pdf/media-news/Paxil-CR-and-Paxil-Adult-Suicide.pdf. Accessed July 25, 2012.

33. Available at: http://abcnews.go.com/Business/wireStory/report-jj-pay-22b-risperdal-settlement-16815635. Accessed July 25, 2012.

34. Available at: http://www.pdrhealth.com/drugs/risperdal. Accessed July 25, 2012.

A Tragic Miscarriage of Justice: We Must Convince the President to Release Jay Kimball

B ACK IN THE YEAR 2004, we dedicated an issue of *Life Extension Magazine®* to the growing threat of wrongful prosecutions that were not based on real "crimes." These prosecutions are instead instigated to serve private business interests, sometimes by pharmaceutical companies that pay "investigators" to find ways to destroy their small competitors. With their enormous political influence, drug companies use these private investigations to persuade the federal government to arrest smaller competitors. The result is that innovative companies offering superior medications at lower prices are destroyed. Pharmaceutical companies financially flourish, while consumers and the healthcare system of the United States collapses under the weight of this relentless corruption.

The most egregious example of prosecutorial misconduct occurred in 2000, when a man named Jay Kimball was sentenced to 13 years in jail for exporting a lower cost liquid deprenyl that may have been superior to the deprenyl tablets being sold for obscenely high prices in the US. The company making the deprenyl tablets launched a massive "private" investigation against Jay Kimball, and then turned their report over to the FDA and Justice Department. Contrary to the 100,000 Americans who die each year from Big Pharma's fraudulently approved drugs, nothing in the private report suggested anyone was harmed by Jay's products. Jay was nonetheless arrested on technical violations of pharmaceutical "export" laws and punished with such a draconian sentence that he may not leave prison alive.

DEPRENYL MAY BE AN ANTI-AGING DRUG

Deprenyl is a drug the FDA approved to treat early-stage Parkinson's disease. It had long before been used throughout Europe. Deprenyl enhances and prolongs the anti-Parkinson effects of standard drugs like L-dopa. Deprenyl has also demonstrated intriguing anti-aging properties.[1-4] According to one study, rats treated with relatively low doses of deprenyl lived up to 38% longer than the control group.[1]

In humans prior to age 45, dopamine levels remain fairly stable. After that, dopamine in the human brain decreases by about 13% each decade. When the dopamine content in the brain reaches about 30% of normal, Parkinson's symptoms may be present.[5] When levels reach 10% of normal, death ensues.[5] This has led to the hypothesis that if we live long enough, we will all develop Parkinson's symptoms due to dopamine depletion in our brains.[1]

Monoamineoxidase B (MAO-B) is an enzyme in the brain that degrades neurotransmitters like dopamine. As humans age, MAO-B levels increase and degrade precious dopamine and other neurotransmitters. Deprenyl is a selective inhibitor of MAO-B.[6] As little as 5 mg twice a week of deprenyl is all aging humans may need to maintain their dopamine at youthful levels.[5] Not only may deprenyl help prevent degenerative brain diseases, but it can also improve the quality of life, as evidenced by increased "mounting frequency" in old male rats treated with deprenyl compared to untreated controls.[5,7-10] Dopamine is a primary "feel good" neurotransmitter that progressively depletes after age 45 in humans.[5] Restoring dopamine levels using low-dose deprenyl (5 mg twice a week) may help aging humans regain some of their youthful sense of well-being.

JAY KIMBALL'S LIQUID DEPRENYL

Deprenyl is now a generic, but when the patent was in force, it sold for a lot of money. Because of the inefficient regulatory environment that limits free-market competition, generic deprenyl costs about the same now as when it was covered under a patent. Jay Kimball had developed a purified liquid deprenyl that he claimed was superior to the outlandishly priced tablets the FDA had approved for Parkinson's patients.[11]

Jay first started selling his liquid deprenyl over-the-counter in the United States. When the FDA ordered him to stop, he capitulated, as his small company lacked the resources to take on the FDA (and Big Pharma) in court. Jay continued, however, to export his liquid deprenyl to other countries.[12] You might ask, what is wrong with exporting medicines to other countries? It turns out that unless the FDA first approves the export, even sending a medication to other countries is "illegal."

PHARMACEUTICAL COMPANY DESTROYS JAY KIMBALL

The pharmaceutical company that sold deprenyl tablets became outraged when Americans who wanted Jay's purportedly superior liquid deprenyl began ordering it from other countries. That is when Jay got into big trouble. The company making deprenyl tablets did not like the low-priced competition, so it ran to the FDA demanding that Jay Kimball be stopped. The FDA did not move fast enough to suit the drug company, so it hired a private detective agency to conduct a criminal investigation independent of the government. The private detectives did a superb job of documenting that Jay was indeed shipping deprenyl to other countries. This file was turned over to the FDA, which used the information supplied by the private investigators to raid Jay Kimball's premises and eventually indict him on numerous criminal counts. There were no victims of Jay Kimball's actions, just violations of FDA "export" regulations.

What happened after Jay was indicted is so unprecedented that few attorneys believe the story until they read it. Just from watching TV, most Americans are aware that defendants are entitled to an attorney and that if they cannot afford one, an attorney will be appointed and paid for by the government. In fact, the government is often quite generous in providing a free attorney for violent street criminals. If you murder someone, the government will sometimes pay an expert criminal defense attorney huge fees so that the "incompetent counsel" argument cannot be used to overturn a death-penalty sentence. Jay did not kill or injure anyone, but he was denied an attorney for his trial. Jay's problem was that he was not indigent, as are most street criminals. Jay had some money to feed his wife and then 13-year-old son and to provide housing for them. The federal government demanded that Jay liquidate all of his assets to pay for an attorney, or else represent himself in court. That would have meant that his wife and son would have to live on the street.

The federal prosecutors offered him a relatively lenient sentence if he pleaded guilty, but Jay defiantly stated that he had not harmed anyone and did not believe he did anything wrong. Jay was told that if he did not plead guilty, he faced up to 3 years in prison if convicted. Jay pleaded for an attorney, but since he was not flat broke, the government would not pay for one. Jay thus had to represent himself in court against the federal prosecutors, the FDA, and the drug company's private detectives. Having never practiced law, Jay did an abysmal job of defending himself and managed to get the judge to despise him in the process. After the jury found Jay guilty, the judge sentenced him to an astounding 13 years in jail, citing Jay's conduct in trial as a reason to add 10 years to what had been a maximum three-year imprisonment.

HEALTH FREEDOM ACTIVISTS TRY TO HELP

When news spread that Jay Kimball was sentenced to 13 years in jail for FDA violations that had harmed no one, the health freedom community was outraged. Jay was denied the basic right to have an attorney represent him, and then was sentenced to 10 years beyond the maximum sentence he was told he would face prior to trial. Federal rules mandate that defendants be told their maximum prison sentence exposure in order to determine whether a guilty plea is appropriate. While Jay had no legal resources to fight with during his trial, donations poured in after his conviction. An appeal was filed seeking to overturn the

10 additional years the judge had arbitrarily and unjustly imposed on him. Despite the best efforts of one of the nation's leading criminal defense firms, the appeal was denied (as most are nowadays).

Jay made it clear to the judge that he was a political dissident and did not recognize the FDA's authority over him. Jay had become the embodiment of a "political prisoner." As is the case in all police-state countries, this meant he would be sent to the harshest jails the Bureau of Prisons could find. He endured filthy county jails in the beginning and then was sent to one of the worst jails (in Belle Glade, FL), where third-world-like squalor breeds infectious diseases among prisoners. Jay contracted traumatic injuries at the hands of guards and infectious diseases that almost killed him. Medical treatment was repeatedly denied.

When the government identifies a political dissident, the punishment often greatly exceeds that of a common street criminal. After all, a dissident dares challenge the very authority of the government itself. An example of this barbaric behavior was Saddam Hussein, who jailed those who committed street crimes but summarily executed those suspected of questioning his absolute authority. The same was true of Adolf Hitler's death camps. Eleven million people were murdered in the Nazi death camps. Six million of those were Jews, with the remainder consisting of unpopular ethnic groups, gypsies, homosexuals, those with physical or mental disabilities, and political dissidents.

Update (2017)

Jay Kimball was released from federal prison in June of 2015 after serving the entirety of his sentence. During the time of his incarceration, both his wife and daughter died from breast cancer.

CHALLENGES WE HAVE CONFRONTED

It has taken us years to get to this point where we can effectively rally health freedom activists to petition the President of the United States to release Jay Kimball. Jay has not made it easy as he has up till now refused to allow us to petition for commutation of sentence. Jay instead relentlessly filed appeals showing in meticulous detail the wrongful nature of his conviction and the illegality of the 13-year sentence.

While imprisoned, Jay's wife developed serious health problems. Jay made a monumental mistake of escaping prison in an attempt to save his wife's life. After Jay developed his own health problems and checked into a hospital using his Medicare account number, he was re-arrested (but not prosecuted for escape). His wife and daughter died afterwards from metastatic breast cancer. His son has not been able to shake off the depression inflicted when his father was taken away at a young age (13 years).

The carnage inflicted on Jay Kimball and his family by this miscarriage of justice defies words. When I first wrote about the plight of Jay Kimball in 2004, some members wrote and assumed I was trying to liberate him because he was a "friend" of mine. That is a categorically false assumption. Jay Kimball has been victimized by an out-of-control criminal justice system to serve the financial wishes of a pharmaceutical company. I am not the kind of person who can sit back and watch the government horrifically trample an individual's rights and do nothing about it.

References

1. Knoll J. Antiaging compounds: (-)deprenyl (selegeline) and (-)1-(benzofuran-2-yl)-2-propylaminopentane, [(-)BPAP], a selective highly potent enhancer of the impulse propagation mediated release of catecholamin. *CNS Drug Rev.* 2001 Fall;7(3):317–45.

2. Dalló J, Köles L. Longevity treatment with (-)deprenyl in female rats: effect on copulatory activity and lifespan. *Acta Physiol Hung.* 1996;84(3):277–8.

3. Kitani K, Kanai S, Carrillo MC, Ivy GO. (-)Deprenyl increases the life span as well as activities of superoxide dismutase and catalase but not of glutathione peroxidase in selective brain regions in Fischer rats. *Ann N Y Acad Sci.* 1994 Jun 30;717:60–71.

4. Freisleben HJ, Lehr F, Fuchs J. Lifespan of immunosuppressed NMRI-mice is increased by deprenyl. *J Neural Transm Suppl.* 1994; 41:231–6.

5. Knoll J. (-)Deprenyl-medication: A strategy to modulate the age-related decline of the striatal dopaminergic system. *J Am Geriatr Soc.* August 1992;40(8): 839–47.

6. Magyar K, Knoll J. Selective inhibition of the "B form" of monoamine oxidase. *Pol J Pharmacol Pharm.* 1977 May-Jun;29(3):233–46.

7. Available at: http://www.lmreview.com/articles/view/an-interview-with-joseph-knoll-md/. Accessed February 8, 2012.

8. Knoll J, Dallo J, Yen TT. Striatal dopamine, sexual activity and lifespan. Longevity of rats treated with (-)deprenyl. *Life Sci.* 1989;45(6):525–31.

9. Gelowitz DL, Richardson JS, Wishart TB, et al. Chronic L-deprenyl or L-amphetamine: equal cognitive enhancement, unequal MAO inhibition. *Pharmacol Biochem Behav.* 1994 Jan;47(1):41–5.

10. Brandeis R, Sapir M, Kapon Y, et al. Improvement of cognitive function by MAO-B inhibitor L-deprenyl in aged rats. 1: *Pharmacol Biochem Behav*. 1991 Jun;39(2):297–304.

11. Available at: http://proliberty.com/observer/20021102. htm. Accessed February 22, 2012.

12. Available at: http://www.iahf.com/free_jay/20001127.html. Accessed February 24, 2012.

Healthcare Crisis:
Can the System Survive?

Healthcare has become a major political and economic issue as medical costs have skyrocketed over the past several decades. "Managed Care" has taken decisions away from doctors and placed them in the hands of insurance companies closely allied with government officials. Private insurers reap profits while government-subsidized plans strain the already overburdened federal and state coffers. Meanwhile, bureaucratic obstacles combine with over-regulated access to treatments with the ultimate result of increased suffering and preventable deaths. What can consumers do? This chapter points out some of the worst failures in the current system and urges citizens to reach out to their representatives in Congress and demand much-needed reform.

Collapsing within Itself

D O YOU REMEMBER when your employer paid 100% of health insurance premiums for you and your family? This free health insurance was widely available in the 1980s and usually covered every medical expense. Back in those days, you did not read about healthcare costs bankrupting individuals, municipalities, corporations, and potentially the federal government. In the 1980s, we at Life Extension® were a lone voice warning of economic turmoil unless medicine was radically deregulated. The government's response to our free-market approach was multiple seizures of products and relentless attempts to jail us. This was done at the behest of those in the mainstream who did not want their government-protected profit machine interfered with.

Move forward 37 years, and exorbitant healthcare costs dominate the financial news. Politicians are desperately trying to figure a way out of a crisis their predecessors created. You may wonder why no one has come up with a real-world solution. Omitted from the debate are the monopolistic pricing powers that regulations bestow to healthcare providers. These regulations (restrictions) preclude innovative competitors from entering the market, while creating mounds of burdensome bureaucracy. Consumers pay for these regulations in the form of high prices, shortages, long waits, side effects, and inferior care.

Inherent inefficiencies within the former Soviet Union led to it collapsing within itself. These same ineptitudes exist with government-regulated medicine in the United States. As we have exposed for 37 consecutive years, the cost of providing quality healthcare is a fraction of what is charged to individuals, insurance companies, and government programs by industries protected by authoritarian edict. Our solution is quite simple. Tear down the regulatory barriers that cause medical costs to be so grossly inflated, and what appears to be a permanent healthcare cost crisis will disappear into the history books.

The media does some accurate reporting about outlandish medical prices, but the public quickly forgets the story. So we did some searching to see how many articles exposing medical-related price gouging we could find. The number was astronomical. When one looks at the magnitude of medical price gouging, and how widespread it is, the reason that healthcare is today's leading political issue becomes brutally apparent. The underlying causes of this financial catastrophe are antiquated regulatory barriers that impede the introduction of more cost-effective ways of delivering better medical care to consumers. These senseless regulatory barriers enable hyperinflated prices since those offering superior medicine at lower prices are not allowed in. What Life Extension® predicted in the 1980s is happening before your eyes. Healthcare costs are spiraling beyond the affordability of the private and public sectors combined.

MARKUPS BEYOND COMPREHENSION

A woman named Jeanne Pinder experienced medical price gouging first hand and uncovered numbers that even startled me.[1] What caused her to be curious was an anesthesia bill for $6,000 from one hospital that was three-times higher than the anesthesia bill from another hospital in the same time-frame. She then questioned why an anti-nausea drug (ondan-setron) was billed by the hospital at $1,419. Jeanne found that the price of ondansetron from a local drug supplier was only $2.49. This indicated the hospital had marked up the price of this one drug by 569 times! Jeanne then did some meticulous research to find out what various insurance plans would pay for ondansetron. For the same drug Jeanne was billed $1,419, the following insurance programs would pay:

Veterans Administration	$15.76
Michigan Blue Cross Blue Shield	$17.60
Medicare	$24.36

The hospital charged $1,419 for a drug that cost less than $3 to buy. Jeanne's investigation provides a real-world example of why healthcare costs have exploded beyond any real-world ability to afford.

Next time you're told more money has to come out of your paycheck or pension to cover increased medical insurance premiums, or your private insurance rates go up, under-stand this is a facade designed to enrich the chosen few in the entrenched medical establishment. It has no basis in economic reality.

NEW YORK TIMES EXPOSES EGREGIOUS MARKUPS

The *New York Times* published an article last year titled "How to Charge $546 for Six Liters of Saltwater."[2] This inves-tigative report looked at what the manufacturer's price was for saline IV solution and what hospitals billed to patients or their insurance carrier. It turned out that some of the patients' bills included markups of 100 to 200 times over the manufacturer's price, not counting separate charges for the administration of the IV solution.

How did the *New York Times* find out the saline cost? Manufacturers are required to report such prices annually to the federal government, which bases Medicare payments on the average national price plus 6%. The limit Medicare would pay for one liter bag of normal saline was $1.07 last year. Yet a bill from a New York hospital charged a private insurance company $91 for a bag of saline that cost the hospital just 86 cents. What consumers forget is that private insurance companies hike insurance premiums based on these inflated drug charges.

CORRUPT LOBBYING CAUSES ASTHMA DRUG PRICE TO SOAR

When an off-patent asthma drug went back on-patent, its price soared from $15 to $100.[3] The name of this old-line drug is albuterol, and it is one of the most common asthma medications used. The way this off-patent asthma drug got back on-patent provides a startling look into the insidious lobbying schemes behind today's inflated drug prices.[3,4]

In order for albuterol to be readily inhaled into the bronchi, it requires a propellant. The propellant in all albuterol drugs was CFC (chlorofluorocarbon). CFC is the ozone-depleting agent that used to spew out of air conditioners, refrigerators, aerosol sprays, and many kinds of industrial equipment. CFC was banned from virtually all uses, but it was still permitted to be used in the small amounts contained in drugs like asthma inhalers until late last year.[5] Pharmaceutical companies that lost patents on medications that used CFC wanted to regain a monopoly on this lucrative market. So they went to the extreme length of contributing $520,000 to a supposed environmental protection group to lobby the FDA to remove CFC from all drugs. This consortium also aggressively developed patented combinations of albuterol and other inhalants with new propellants that won FDA approval.[6]

This nefarious lobbying effort paid off. In 2005, the FDA approved an outright ban on many CFC-based inhalers starting in 2009.[7] Subsequent bans took effect on other CFC drugs.[7,8] Bear in mind that the consortium behind this lobbying scheme consisted of the same companies selling CFC-propelled drugs. They were effectively lobbying the FDA to ban their own drugs so they could monopolize the market with the new propellant versions they were patenting.[6] CFC was the most effective medical propellant and according to some scientists, when compared to global CFC emissions, the tiny quantity used in inhalers posed no significant negative impact on the ozone layer.[6] The payoff for this deceptive lobbying campaign was a 6-fold increase in the price that could be charged for the new patented albuterol that was inferior to the previous CFC version in delivering the drug to suffocating asthmatics.[8]

Schemes like this to rip off consumers are not exceptions. They are customary business practices of companies that routinely deceive the courts, Congress, and the FDA to deny generic competitors access to the market and stomp out the introduction of new medical products that could save lives and lower healthcare costs. Do you see why there is no real healthcare cost crisis? There is instead a crooked marketplace dominated by lobbyists who use the government's regulatory barriers to gouge the public with monopolistic prices.

ANALOGIZING THIS TO GAS PRICES

Just imagine if Exxon® wanted to monopolize the gasoline market and patented a less-efficient way of refining crude oil into gasoline. Then imagine Exxon® funds a fake environmental group to lobby the EPA (Environmental Protection Agency) to ban currently used refining methods. Exxon® would then monopolize the market with its patented refining method and be able to increase the retail price of gasoline from $3 a gallon to let's say $18—the same 6-fold increase that occurred with albuterol. This would force consumers to spend over $300 to fill their tank. Since most people cannot afford a $300 gas tank fill, Exxon® would need to emulate pharmaceutical companies and persuade the government to use tax dollars to subsidize their artificially inflated prices. This would force the government to set up a special website to determine which Americans were eligible for gasoline subsidies based on individual income levels.

Do you see what a mess this would create? There is no way that government could afford to subsidize these artificially inflated gas prices, nor could companies do so for their employees or unions for their members. Yet this is exactly what is happening with conventional medical costs. Prices are being corruptly inflated, and all Congress does is bicker as to who is going to pay it. The harsh fact is that no one can afford to keep paying for something that is corruptly priced far beyond its free-market value. The fallout from this occurs before our eyes with the pending insolvencies of Medicare, Medicaid, municipal health plans, along with large swaths of the American economic landscape, including the post office.

THIS CATASTROPHE IS AVOIDABLE

Medical care is not a luxury. It becomes a necessity when one falls ill. Medical care is so essential that hundreds of different state and federal government programs have been created to regulate and pay for it. Yet many of these government programs encourage fraud and force inefficiencies. The end result has become price gouging so severe that medical care has become unaffordable to society as a whole. By way of example, the average annual cost per household for healthcare is around $20,000.[9] The average household, however, does not earn enough to part with $20,000, so no tax and redistribution system is ever going to work in the long run.

Common sense deregulation, on the other hand, would force vast improvements in healthcare while dramatically lowering costs. Compare this to the electronic industry, which has seen exponential technological enhancements, but constantly plummeting prices. If these kinds of advances had ever been translated to the medical arena, cures for virtually every degenerative disease would likely have already occurred.

FALLACY OF AFFORDABLE CARE ACT

Proponents of government-subsidized healthcare fail to realize the inflationary impact it has on healthcare prices.[10-12] When the Medicare Modernization and Prescription Drug Act of 2003 was passed, it gave pharmaceutical companies free rein to charge the federal government full retail price on prescription drugs covered by the Act.[13] It should be no surprise that the Medicare Modernization and Prescription Drug Act of 2003 was written and pushed into law by pharmaceutical lobbyists.

The Affordable Care Act passed in 2010 is deceptively named. Premiums and co-pays for typical people are high, while annual deductibles are exorbitant.[14-16] My private health insurance premium in 1982 was only $780 per year and paid full expenses for any hospital facility I chose in the

United States. My deductible was virtually non-existent. The Affordable Care Act restricts where policy holders can get treatment, which can be a problem when a superior therapy is located outside one's community hospital network. Under the current so-called "Affordable" Care Act, young people today are paying around $3,000 a year in premiums for basic health insurance and are faced with annual deductibles of over $5,000![17,18] A significant percentage of the population does not have $5,000–$6,000 to cover their annual deductible, meaning the government-mandated insurance premiums they pay are often of little real-world value.

The more accurately defined "Unaffordable Care Act" has spawned fierce debate. When you see politicians attacking each other over how to best fund soaring sick-care costs, remember that there is no real-world solution as long as the government grants monopolistic pricing power to conventional medicine. High medical prices would plummet in a deregulated environment, and the need for an "affordable" care act might become obsolete.

WHAT YOU CAN DO

The public is slowly recognizing the disconnection between medical costs and the inflated prices consumers are forced to bear. Media stories exposing over-priced healthcare are seen one day but often forgotten the next. Politicians act oblivious to medical price gouging and can't stop arguing about where the money should come from to fund bloated healthcare costs. If Congress just investigated why American medicine is so expensive, they might understand the need to remove archaic regulatory barriers that underlie the problem.

Five years ago, my book *Pharmocracy* was published for the purpose of exposing the flaws in the current regulatory system that cause healthcare to be so overpriced. I want to encourage members to not waver in this battle and to send a hard copy of *Pharmocracy II* to their Representative and/or two Senators. Rather than sit back and watch our nation financially flounder, contact your legislators and demand reform now.

References

1. Available at: http://clearhealthcosts.com/blog/2010/11/the-1481-drug-markup/. Accessed March 10, 2014.

2. Available at: http://www.nytimes.com/2013/08/27/health/exploring-salines-secret-costs.html?_r=0. Accessed March 10, 2014.

3. Available at: http://www.nytimes.com/2013/10/13/us/the-soaring-cost-of-a-simple-breath.html. Accessed March 10, 2014.

4. Available at: http://www.gpo.gov/fdsys/pkg/CHRG-111hhrg50066/html/CHRG-111hhrg50066.htm. Accessed March 10, 2014.

5. Available at: http://www.fda.gov/newsevents/newsroom/pressannouncements/ucm371901.htm. Accessed March 11, 2014.

6. Available at: http://www.motherjones.com/environment/2011/07/cost-increase-asthma-inhalers-expensive. Accessed March 11, 2014.

7. Available at: http://www.motherjones.com/kevin-drum/2013/10/heres-why-your-asthma-inhaler-costs-so-damn-much. Accessed March 11, 2014.

8. Available at: http://www.fda.gov/Drugs/ResourcesForYou/Consumers/QuestionsAnswers/ucm077808.htm. Accessed March 11, 2014.

9. Available at http://www.money.cnn.com/2012/03/29/pf/healthcare-costs/. Accessed March 11, 2014.

10. Available at: http://bastiat.mises.org/2013/12/how-government-regulations-made-healthcare-so-expensive. Accessed June 2, 2014.

11. Available at: http://www.safehaven.com/article/32015/the-effect-of-the-affordable-care-act-on-medical-care-inflation. Accessed June 2, 2014.

12. Available at:http://www.galen.org/topics/ten-obamacare-predictions-for-2014/. Accessed June 2, 2014.

13. Available at: http://abcnews.go.com/Nightline/story?id=128998. Accessed June 2, 2014.

14. Available at: http://www.humanevents.com/2014/03/19/obamacare-sticker-shock-get-ready-for-your-jacked-up-premiums-to-double-or-even-triple. Accessed June 2, 2014.

15. Available at: http://www.cbsnews.com/news/obamacare-deductibles-deliver-hefty-sticker-shock. Accessed June 2, 2014.

16. Available at: http://www.healthpocket.com/healthcare-research/infostat/2014-obamacare-deductible-out-of-pocket-costs. Accessed June 2, 2014.

17. Available at: http://www.healthpocket.com/healthcare-research/infostat/2014-obamacare-deductible-out-of-pocket-costs. Accessed June 2, 2014.

18. Available at: http://www.forbes.com/sites/jeffreydorfman/2013/10/31/the-high-costs-of-obamacare-hit-home-for-the-middle-class. Accessed June 2, 2014.

19. Available at: http://www.bloomberg.com/news/2013-11-15/obamacare-deductibles-26-higher-make-cheap-rates-a-risk.html. Accessed June 2, 2014.

Former FDA Commissioner Admits Risk of Bureaucratic Delay

ED KENNEDY WAS DIAGNOSED WITH A BRAIN TUMOR in May 2008. He received the best conventional treatment at Duke University Medical Center, which enabled him to survive until August 2009—a total of 15 months. I'll never forget being told when I was age 14 about a young girl who was dying of a brain tumor. I asked a lot of ignorant questions as to why doctors could not cure it, but no one had any logical answers. That was back in 1968, yet a person stricken today with the most common brain tumor (glioblastoma multiforme) will only live a few miserable months longer than in the past.[1] Over the years, the media has announced the discovery of promising cancer therapies, but most never make it to the clinical testing stage.

We at Life Extension® have been harshly critical of the FDA's drug approval process, arguing that medical innovation has been suffocated by high costs and bureaucratic uncertainties. An increasing number of respected individuals are agreeing that delaying lifesaving therapies can no longer be tolerated, including former FDA Commissioner Andrew von Eschenbach. Dr. von Eschenbach is a former director of the National Cancer Institute and served as FDA Commissioner from 2005 to 2009. He authored an editorial published in the *Wall Street Journal* that was critical of the FDA's ability to evaluate and approve new life-saving therapies.[2] The editorial opened by Dr. von Eschenbach stating:

> We stand on the cusp of a revolution in healthcare. Advances in molecular medicine will allow us to develop powerful new treatments that can cure or even prevent diseases like Alzheimer's and cancer. What's missing . . . is a modernized Food and Drug Administration that can rapidly and efficiently bring new discoveries to patients.[2]

Dr. von Eschenbach cited current FDA Commissioner Margaret Hamburg's concession before Congress that, "The FDA is relying on 20th century regulatory science to evaluate 21st century medical products."[3] The most compelling arguments Dr. von Eschenbach made for meaningful reform were:

> The FDA should approve drugs based on safety and leave efficacy testing for post-market studies. Congress can ensure that the FDA serves as a bridge— not a barrier—to cutting-edge technologies.[2]

Said differently, once a potentially effective therapy has been cleared for safety, it should be made immediately available to human beings who will otherwise suffer and die. Brain tumor patients, for example, don't have years to wait for FDA-mandated efficacy studies. They need rapid access to new therapies that offer some hope of saving their lives.

DR. VON ESCHENBACH DISCUSSES REGENERATIVE MEDICINE

Dr. von Eschenbach wrote:

> Breakthrough technologies deserve a breakthrough in the way the FDA evaluates them. Take regenerative medicine. If a company can grow cells that repair the retina in a lab, patients who've been blinded by macular degeneration shouldn't have to wait years while the FDA asks the company to complete laborious clinical trials proving efficacy. Instead, after proof of concept and safety testing, the product could be approved for marketing with every eligible patient entered in a registry so the company and the FDA can establish efficacy through post-market studies.[4]

This common sense approach has been advocated by Life Extension® for more than 30 years. It's refreshing to see a former FDA Commissioner concur.

BRIDGING THE FDA'S "DEATH VALLEY"

Newly diagnosed cancer patients are usually given several treatment choices, all laden with guaranteed side effects with no promise of a cure or even a significant remission. For most types of cancer, progress has been excruciatingly slow, even though there are more scientific studies being published about cancer now than at any time in human history. The term "death valley" is increasingly being used to describe the gap that separates what is discovered in the scientific setting from what actually makes it into patients' bodies. The sad fact is there are so many bureaucratic roadblocks that potentially effective therapies aren't making it out of the laboratory setting. The high costs of conducting human efficacy trials deny smaller companies equal opportunity to bring what may be superior medications to market. Dr. von Eschenbach's proposal to allow new therapies on the market as soon as safety is established would liberate many promising therapies currently trapped in the FDA's oppressive quagmire.

WHO DOES NOT WANT FASTER APPROVAL?

There are those who financially benefit by maintaining the current system that requires enormous capital expenditures and many years of delay before new therapies are approved. Large pharmaceutical companies enjoy a quasi-monopoly on the development of new drugs because virtually no one else can afford the gargantuan costs of FDA approval. When small companies make a medical discovery, pharmaceutical giants often buy out the technology because smaller companies lack the resources to afford currently mandated efficacy studies.

There's also the issue of the enormous profitability on existing therapies. Just look at the melanoma drug called Yervoy made by Bristol Myers Squib. It costs $120,000 for this treatment that only extends survival in advanced melanoma patients an average of 108 days.[5] It is in the economic interests of Bristol Myers Squib that no other melanoma therapy be approved for the next 20 years so they can collect $120,000 from every melanoma patient who is not cured in the early stage. Pharmaceutical giants stand to earn enormous profits as long as it costs so much to comply with FDA efficacy requirements that competition from superior therapies is stifled.

WHERE WE DON'T AGREE WITH DR. VON ESCHENBACH

There is a misconception in the mainstream that if the FDA were given more resources, that it could properly do its job.

This fallacy was exposed in a report the FDA commissioned wherein it revealed that the FDA had systemic internal flaws that could not be corrected by the mere input of more money.[6] While Dr. von Eschenbach emphasizes the need to modernize the FDA "from the bottom up" to include a "comprehensive external review of the agency's regulatory processes,"[7] the track record of federal agencies improving themselves is abysmal, especially with powerful special interests like pharmaceutical companies vehemently opposing any change.

WHY "EFFICACY" IS SOMETIMES MORE IMPORTANT THAN "SAFETY"

The public rightfully fears the risks posed by unsafe drugs, and we at Life Extension® have written many exposés on dangerous medicines the FDA should never have approved. Yet the reality is that even the worst side-effect-prone drugs only affect a minority of patients. When it comes to treating terminal diseases like Alzheimer's and certain cancers, efficacy becomes paramount to safety because these patients will die unless an experimental therapy happens to work for them. So restricting promising therapies to only those with proven safety will continue to condemn certain Americans to guaranteed death, which is why some patients need even earlier access to experimental treatments than what Dr. von Eschenbach proposes.

THE FDA HAS LONG DELAYED LIFE-SAVING DRUGS

The current and former Commissioners of the FDA state that the FDA is incapable of approving 21st century technologies in a timely fashion. What they may not know is that the FDA delayed approval of life-saving therapies for much of the 20th century. A chilling example is that of propranolol, a beta-blocker that saves the lives of tens of thousands of Americans each year. Propranolol was used in Europe many years before the FDA approved it in the US.[8,9] If you multiply the number of lives that could have been saved each year if US patients had gained access to propranolol—times the multi-year delay—the total number exceeds 30,000 Americans who needlessly died because of the FDA's delay in approving this ONE drug.[9]

The anti-diabetic drug metformin was approved in England in 1958, but the FDA did not get around to allowing it in the United States until 1994.[10] Metformin is now the first-line treatment for early-stage diabetes.[11-13] The number of type II diabetics who perished needlessly because they did not have access to metformin is incalculable.

The anti-viral drug ribavirin was used throughout the world in the early 1980s, but FDA did not approve it for use in America until 1998.[14-18] Ribavirin increases the efficacy of interferon in treating hepatitis C. It is a broad-spectrum drug that can eradicate a wide range of lethal viruses, yet Americans died while ribavirin was sold over-the-counter in some countries.

Since the early 1960s, when Congress granted the agency authoritarian new powers, the FDA has functioned as a roadblock that denies Americans access to improved medical therapies. The timeline from when a drug demonstrates safety and the inordinate number of years it takes to gain regulatory approval speaks for itself.

LETHAL CONSEQUENCES OF DENIAL

Politicians are debating a lot of topics right now, but the most important problem facing Americans is not being discussed. Once you or a loved one is diagnosed with a serious disease, all other issues become largely irrelevant. Your only concern is whether there is a non-toxic cure available. That's why it's imperative that free-market reforms are enacted that place the FDA in an advisory role that allows rapid medical progress unimpeded by central government bureaucrats.

In response to Dr. von Eschenbach's editorial, a number of doctors responded with complimentary letters, but emphasized that even more deregulation of FDA authoritarian control is needed to bring about cures for today's killer diseases.[19] Some of these letters exposed how dysfunction and unpredictability at the FDA is precluding vital early-stage scientific research.

The sad fact is that most of the American public remains in a state of denial about the lethal consequences of today's antiquated regulatory structure. This denial turns into harsh reality when one is diagnosed with an illness for which there is no current cure. We at Life Extension® continue our relentless campaign to alert policy makers and the public about the urgent need to accelerate the introduction of new therapies. This can only happen if the major roadblock (i.e., the FDA) is relegated to an advisory role, away from its current dictatorial role. Unlike any other issue, failure to affect meaningful FDA reform will result in millions of Americans needlessly suffering and dying every single year. This is no longer just the opinion of health freedom fighters like me, but also the current and former Commissioners of the FDA!

AS MY ARTICLE WAS GOING TO PRESS . . .

A White House advisory body on September 25, 2012, unveiled a plan to increase the number of new prescription drugs that go on the market each year by more quickly approving drugs to treat high-risk patients. The President's Council of Advisors on Science and Technology urged the FDA to expand its use of faster drug approvals to a wider range of diseases. The council suggested the FDA could begin to approve drugs that may help only a narrow and high-risk patient population, such as people who are morbidly obese, under what the council called "special medical use" approvals. While it is encouraging to see the White House agree with our long-standing position about the lethal consequences of drug delays, these kinds of changes are inadequate to address the cumbersome bureaucracy that impedes scientific discoveries from reaching the clinical setting where they are desperately needed by terminally ill humans.

References

1. Henriksson R, Asklund T, Poulsen HS. Impact of therapy on quality of life, neurocognitive function and their correlates in glioblastoma multiforme: a review. *J Neurooncol.* 2011 Sep;104(3):639–46. Epub 2011 Apr 6.

2. Available at: http://online.wsj.com/article/SB1000142405 29702036460045772154033 99350874.html. Accessed on July 16, 2012.

3. Available at: http://www.fda.gov/downloads/AboutFDA/ ReportsManualsForms/Reports/BudgetReports/ UCM244196.pdf. Accessed April 4, 2012.

4. Available at: http://www.policymed.com/2012/04/former-fda-commissioner-calls-for-updated-systems-and-more-education-for-fda.html. Accessed April 10, 2012.

5. Available at: http://www.nytimes.com/2011/03/26/ business/26drug.html?_r=1. Accessed April 10, 2012.

6. Available at: http://www.fda.gov/ohrms/dockets/AC/07/ briefing/2007-4329b_02_01_FDA%20Report%20on%20 Science%20and%20Technology.pdf. Accessed April 10, 2012.

7. Available at: http://eyewiretoday.com/view.asp?20120214-wsj_the_fda_should_approve_drugs_based_on_safety_and_

leave_efficacy_testing_for_post-market_studies. Accessed July 16, 2012.

8. Available at: http://www.fdareview.org/harm.shtml. Accessed April 12, 2012.

9. Available at: http://www.isil.org/resources/lit/death-regulation. html. Accessed April 12, 2012.

10. Available at: http://onlinelibrary.wiley.com/doi/10.1111/ j.1464-5491.2011.03469.x/pdf. Accessed April 12, 2012.

11. Bennett WL, Maruthur NM, Singh S, et al. Comparative effectiveness and safety of medications for type 2 diabetes: an update including new drugs and 2-drug combinations. *Ann Intern Med*. 2011 May 3;154(9):602–13. Epub 2011 Mar 14.

12. Available at: http://care.diabetesjournals.org/content/32/ Supplement_1/S13.full. Accessed April 13, 2012.

13. Available at: http://www.ncbi.nlm.nih.gov/books/NBK55754/. Accessed July 16, 2012.

14. Knight V, McClung HW, Wilson SZ, Waters BK, Quarles JM, Cameron RW, Greggs SE, Zerwas JM, Couch RB. Ribavirin small-particle aerosol treatment of influenza. *Lancet*. 1981 Oct 31;2(8253):945–9.

15. Davis GL, Balart LA, Schiff ER, et al. Treatment of chronic hepatitis C with recombinant interferon alfa. A multicenter randomized, controlled trial. Hepatitis Interventional Therapy Group. *N Engl J Med*. 1989 Nov 30;321(22):1501–6.

16. Reichard O, Norkrans G, Frydén A, Braconier JH, Sönnerborg A, Weiland O. Randomised, double-blind, placebo-controlled trial of interferon alpha-2b with and without ribavirin for chronic hepatitis C. The Swedish Study Group. *Lancet*. 1998 Jan 10;351(9096):83–7.

17. de Lédinghen V, Trimoulet P, Winnock M, et al; French Multicenter Study Group. Daily or three times per week interferon alpha-2b in combination with ribavirin or interferon alone for the treatment of patients with chronic hepatitis

C not responding to previous interferon alone. *J Hepatol.* 2002 Jun;36(6):819–26.

18. Ali S, Nazir G, Khan SA, Iram S, Fatima F. Comparative therapeutic response to pegylated interferon plus ribavirin versus interferon alpha-2b in chronic hepatitis C patients. *J Ayub Med Coll Abbottabad.* 2010 Oct-Dec;22(4):127–30.

19. Available at: http://online.wsj.com/article/SB10001424052 970204792404577229641193886650.html. Accessed July 16, 2012.

How Regulation of Medicine Is Bankrupting the United States and What Congress Can Do to Stop It

EVEN COMPOUNDED TESTOSTERONE COSTS TOO MUCH

FDA REGULATIONS PROHIBIT compounding pharmacies from making production-scale batches of popular drugs. Each compounded drug must be individually formulated by a licensed pharmacist. The result is that the labor involved in making a compounded drug comprises more than what the active ingredient costs. But there are additional regulations that add even greater costs.

Consumers require a prescription to buy compounded testosterone just like they do with FDA-approved testosterone. While competent physician supervision can enhance the safety and efficacy of a testosterone replacement program, the frank reality is that the majority of prescriptions for drugs like AndroGel® are not prescribed by physicians who understand how to optimally manage hormone replacement in men. Seldom are estrogen levels monitored to protect against estrogen overload that can occur when too much testosterone converts (aromatizes) into estrogen in an aging man's body.[41,42] An advantage with compounded testosterone is that if a physician knows how to write a prescription for it, they often have received training on follow-up monitoring. Compounded testosterone cream can be obtained for less than $50 a month, compared to almost $200 for AndroGel®. Either form can contain the same amount of bioidentical testosterone. Compounded testosterone cream is 91% less expensive than FDA-protected drugs, yet compounded testosterone is still twice as expensive as it needs to be because of governmental over-regulation.

In dealing with runaway healthcare costs, a solution is to make drugs like testosterone available to men over age 40 without the need of a doctor's visit. There have been companies that have physicians review blood tests over the phone and prescribe testosterone, but FDA and state licensing boards have shut many of these down.[43] Corrupt regulations ensure that efficiencies that would slash healthcare cost (at the expense of pharmaceutical profits) are outlawed.

SIMPLE SOLUTION TO AVERT ECONOMIC RUINATION

Life Extension® initiated a petition drive back in the 1980s to allow individual Americans to "opt-out" of the FDA's regulatory umbrella. Our rationale was that this would provide consumers with more advanced treatments at lower prices. Hundreds of our enlightened members petitioned, requesting liberation from the FDA stranglehold. The public, Congress, and media were apathetic at that time. The FDA was far from lethargic. They responded to our petition in a way that resembled an angry hornet's nest when disturbed (or how some dictators respond to street protestors). The notion that we dared challenge the FDA's absolute authority resulted in years of legal battles in which the FDA did everything in its power to destroy us.[44]

Move forward to today, and the political climate has turned around. The healthcare cost crisis we long ago predicted has evolved into a harsh reality no one can ignore. It is mathematically impossible to solve it by forcing one group to pay regulated medicine's inflated costs. The only salvation is the free-market reforms we long ago drafted. Our proposal is quite simple. Amend the law to allow good manufacturing practice (GMP) certified facilities to produce generic prescription drugs that do not undergo the excessive regulatory hurdles that force consumers to pay egregiously inflated prices. To alert consumers when they are getting a generic whose manufacturing is not as heavily regulated as it is currently, the law would mandate that the label of these less-regulated generic drugs clearly states:

> This is not an FDA-approved manufactured generic drug and may be ineffective and potentially dangerous. This drug is NOT manufactured under the same standards required for an FDA-approved generic drug. Purchase this drug at your own risk.

By allowing the sale of these less costly generics, consumers will have a choice as to what companies they choose to trust.

Equally important in our proposals is allowing consumers to be told about the off-label benefits of prescription drugs, such as the extensive body of evidence that metformin may help prevent type 2 diabetes[45,46] (and not just treat it) and that metformin may also prevent and help treat certain cancers.[47-54]

A concern critics raise regarding this free-market solution is safety. Who will protect consumers from poorly made generic drugs, they ask? First of all, there will be the same regulation of these drugs as there is with GMP-certified supplement makers. FDA inspectors will visit facilities, take sample products, and assay to ensure potency of active ingredient and dissolution. Laboratories that fail to make products that meet label claims would face civil and criminal penalties from the government. Secondly, there is no incentive not to provide the full potency of active ingredient in these less regulated generic drugs. The price of the active ingredients makes up such a small percentage of the overall cost that a manufacturer would be idiotic to scrimp on potency.[55]

Companies that foolishly make inferior generics will be viciously exposed by the media, along with the FDA, consumer protection groups, and even prescribing physicians, who will be suspicious if a drug is not working as it is supposed to. Companies producing inferior products will be quickly driven from the marketplace as consumers who choose to purchase these lower-cost generics will seek out laboratories that have reputations for making flawless products. Substandard companies would not only be castigated in the public's eye, but face civil litigation from customers who bought the defective generics. When one considers that GMP-certified manufacturing plants can cost hundreds of millions to set up, a company would guarantee itself future insolvency if it failed to produce generic drugs that met minimum standards.

PHARMACEUTICAL COMPANY PROPAGANDA

No matter how many facts show that free-market generic drugs can be made safe, there are alarmists who believe that even if one person suffers a serious adverse event because of a lower-cost generic drug, then the law should not be amended to allow the sale of these less regulated products. What few understand is that enabling lower-cost drugs to be sold might reduce the number of poorly made drugs. The reason is that prescription drug counterfeiting is a major issue today.[56] Drugs are counterfeited because they are so expensive. Yet in the free-market environment we espouse, a month's supply of a popular cholesterol-lowering drug like simvastatin would sell for only $3. It is difficult to imagine anyone profiting by counterfeiting it. So amending the law to enable these super low-cost drugs to be sold might reduce the counterfeiting that exists right now.

Another reason these less regulated generics will do far more good than harm is that people who need them to live will be able to afford them. The media has reported on heart-wrenching stories of destitute people who are unable to pay for their prescription drugs. They either do without or take a less-than-optimal dose. The availability of these free-market generics will enable virtually anyone to be able to afford their medications.

Those who think generic drugs are safe today should be aware of isolated instances when improperly made active ingredients make it into prescription drugs sold in US pharmacies. These defective ingredients often emanate from FDA-approved manufacturers in China and India. The FDA gives false assurances that these government-approved laboratories are safe. The reality is that the FDA can only inspect each Chinese drug-making factory at best only once every 13 years.[57] So the protection consumers think they have today is a facade. I would feel more comfortable buying generics from a company that had its own inspectors in offshore manufacturing facilities as opposed to relying on meaningless FDA rhetoric.

AS MY ARTICLE WAS BEING FINALIZED . . .

As my article was being finalized, news broke that the FDA had just granted an exclusive monopoly to a company to sell a non-patented progesterone drug that prevents premature births.[58] Healthy women naturally secrete huge amounts of progesterone during pregnancy that helps maintain their uterine lining. To protect against premature births and miscarriages in women at risk, enlightened doctors have for decades prescribed progesterone medications that were made by state-licensed compounding pharmacies. The cost per injection was around $20. By granting orphan drug status to one company (KV Pharmaceutical), FDA rules banned all other forms of progesterone for this indication. The immediate impact was that the cost per injection skyrocketed to $1,500—or as much as $30,000 for a full-term pregnancy.[59] An uprising over this price gouging forced the FDA to back down and state it "does not intend to take enforcement action against pharmacies that compound hydroxy-progesterone caproate."

What the FDA is saying is that while it has the discretion to arrest compounding pharmacists for making this drug, it does not "intend to" do so. After the FDA made this announcement, KV Pharmaceutical reduced the price to $690 per injection—which is still more than 34 times its previous free-market price. It is unclear how private insurance and Medicaid will determine whether to pay $690 per injection for the version FDA rules state is the only one that can be legally sold or continue paying for the much lower-cost compounded version.

Women who are denied access to this drug because of the regulatory quagmire face increased risks they will deliver pre-term babies. In these cases, the costs for intensive neonatology care can run into the hundreds of thousands of dollars per premature-born baby, a price often borne by Medicaid or private insurance. No country on earth can afford this kind of institutionalized corruption, where the chosen few pharmaceutical companies favored by the FDA reap extortionist profits as the nation collapses into a financial abyss. This rare instance in which public backlash forced the FDA to back away from protecting a pharmaceutical company's obscene profit reveals that citizens have the power the save this country from financial Armageddon.

FIGHT BACK AGAINST THIS INSTITUTIONAL CORRUPTION

The United States of America faces a healthcare cost crisis that will render Medicare, Medicaid, and many private insurance plans insolvent. The shocking details about this country's inability to fund future medical costs are no longer confined to the pages of *Life Extension Magazine®*. You are reading about them virtually every day in the mainstream media.[60,61]

When terrorists attacked the United States in 2001, there were patriotic Americans who enlisted in the armed services. Many lost their limbs, their vision, and their lives. No one has to engage in physical combat to save this country from the institutionalized inefficiencies and corruption that plague today's disease-care system.

This book provides irrefutable logic to reform today's broken healthcare system. We believe if enough citizens send *Pharmocracy II* to Congress, that our leaders will be forced to recognize the obvious free-market solutions to today's broken healthcare system. To order copies of *Pharmocracy II* today call 1-800-544-4440.

References

1. Available at: http://www.sciencedaily.com/releases/2009/08/090818182051.htm. Accessed March 24, 2011.

2. Available at: http://www.csmonitor.com/2003/1028/p01s02-usec.html. Accessed March 24, 2011.

3. Available at: https://www.cms.gov/ReportsTrustFunds/downloads/tr2011.pdf. Accessed July 1, 2011.

4. Available at: http://www.gao.gov/financial/fy2010/10frusg.pdf. Accessed March 24, 2011.

5. Available at: http://www.economicsjunkie.com/the-coming-us-tax-receipt-shortfall/. Accessed July 14, 2011.

6. Available at: http://www.whitehouse.gov/the_press_office/remarks-by-the-president-to-a-joint-session-of-congress-on-health-care. Accessed March 24, 2011.

7. Available at: http://waysandmeans.house.gov/News/DocumentSingle.aspx?DocumentID=244984. Accessed July 1, 2011.

8. Available at: http://www.forbes.com/2009/05/14/taxes-social-security-opinions-columnists-medicare.html. Accessed March 24, 2011.

9. Available at: http://www.cms.gov/ReportsTrustFunds/Downloads/2011TRAlternativeScenario.pdf. Accessed July 1, 2011.

10. Available at: http://www.nytimes.com/2011/03/26/business/26drug.html. Accessed June 21, 2011.

11. Available at: http://www.nytimes.com/2008/07/06/health/06avastin.html. Accessed June 21, 2011.

12. Available at: http://www.usatoday.com/yourlife/health/medical/cancer/2010-11-18-provenge-medicare_N.htm. Accessed June 21, 2011.

13. Available at: http://www.glgroup.com/News/If-you-think-health-care-and-Medicare-are-problems-consider-long-term-care-and-Medicaid.-30757.html. Accessed March 24, 2011.

14. Available at: http://www.heritage.org/research/reports/2005/10/the-economic-and-fiscal-effects-of-financing-medicares-unfunded-liabilities. Accessed March 24, 2011.

15. Available at: http://biggovernment.com/publius/2011/07/05/the-compensation-monster-devouring-cities/. Accessed Mar 24, 2011.

16. Available at: http://www.economist.com/node/13983688?story_id=13983688. Accessed March 24, 2011.

17. Available at: http://yourwisdom.yahoo.com/your-health/avastin-cancer-treatment-drug-actually-raises-risk-death-article-acid.html. Accessed March 24, 2011.

18. Available at: http://www.pcrm.org/newsletter/aug10/diabetes_drugs.html. Accessed March 24, 2011.

19. Ranpura V, Hapani S, Wu S. Treatment-related mortality with bevacizumab in cancer patients: a meta-analysis. JAMA. 2011 Feb 2;305(5):487–94.

20. Available at: http://rutherfordtimesonline.com/2010/03/09/the-audacity-of-freedom-government-regulation-of-the-pharmaceutical-industry-harms-more-than-helps. Accessed March 24, 2011

21. Available at: http://www.progressiveradionetwork.com/health-headlines/2010/7/16/special-report-pharmaceutical-profit-big-government-and-bias.html. Accessed March 24, 2011.

22. Available at: http://www.anh-usa.org/access-to-estriol-2/. Accessed March 24, 2011.

23. Available at: http://iacprx.convio.net/site/DocServer/Wyeth_Campaign_Fact_Sheet_0408.pdf?docID=3881&JServSessionIdr004=ibxg9a4i53.app214b. Accessed July 15, 2011.

24. Rossouw JE, Anderson GL, Prentice RL, et al. Risks and benefits of estrogen plus progestin in healthy postmenopausal women: principal results From the Women's Health Initiative randomized controlled trial. JAMA. 2002 Jul 17;288(3):321–33.

25. Slatore CG, Chien JW, Au DH, Satia JA, White E. Lung cancer and hormone replacement therapy: association in the vitamins and lifestyle study. J Clin Oncol. 2010 Mar 20;28(9):1540–6.

26. Cushman M, Kuller LH, Prentice R, et al. Estrogen plus progestin and risk of venous thrombosis. JAMA. 2004 Oct 6;292(13):1573–80.

27. Beral V. Breast cancer and hormone-replacement therapy in the Million Women Study. Lancet. 2003 Aug 9;362(9382):419–27.

28. Anderson GL, Judd HL, Kaunitz AM, et al. Effects of estrogen plus progestin on gynecologic cancers and associated diagnostic procedures: the Women's Health Initiative randomized trial. JAMA. 2003 Oct 1;290(13):1739–48.

29. Manson JE, Hsia J, Johnson KC, et al. Estrogen plus progestin and the risk of coronary heart disease. N Engl J Med. 2003 Aug 7;349(6):523–34.

30. Shumaker SA, Legault C, Rapp SR, et al. Estrogen plus progestin and the incidence of dementia and mild cognitive impairment in postmenopausal women: the Women's Health Initiative Memory Study: a randomized controlled trial. JAMA. 2003 May 28;289(20):2651–62.

31. Chen CL, Weiss NS, Newcomb P, Barlow W, White E. Hormone replacement therapy in relation to breast cancer. JAMA. 2002 Feb 13;287(6):734–41.

32. Nakamura Y, Yogosawa S, Izutani Y, Watanabe H, Otsuji E, Sakai T. A combination of indol-3-carbinol and genistein synergistically induces apoptosis in human colon cancer HT-29 cells by inhibiting Akt phosphorylation and progression of autophagy. Mol Cancer. 2009 Nov 12;8:100.

33. Katdare M, Osborne MP, Telang NT. Inhibition of aberrant proliferation and induction of apoptosis in pre-neoplastic human mammary epithelial cells by natural phytochemicals. Oncol Rep. 1998 Mar-Apr; 5(2):311–5.

34. Available at: http://www.appliedhealth.com/index.php?option=com_content&view=article&id=107071&Itemid=205. Accessed March 25, 2011.

35. Available at: http://www.anh-usa.org/bioidentical-estriol-still-under-threat/. Accessed March 25, 2011.

36. Faloon W. FDA seeks to ban pyridoxamine. *Life Extension Magazine®*. 2009 Jul;15(7):7–12.

37. Available at: http://www.fda.gov/NewsEvents/Newsroom/PressAnnouncements/2008/ucm116832.htm. Accessed March 25, 2011.

38. Available at: http://articles.mercola.com/sites/articles/archive/2011/03/22/betrayal-of-consumers-by-us-supreme-court-gives-total-liability-shield-to-big-pharma.aspx. Accessed March 25, 2011.

39. Available at: http://www.pharmalot.com/2007/04/60_minutes_beats_up_big_pharma/. Accessed March 25, 2011.

40. Faloon W. Startling low testosterone levels in male Life Extension members. *Life Extension Magazine®*. 2010 June; 16(6);7–12.

41. Vermeulen A, Kaufman JM, Goemaere S, van Pottelberg I. Estradiol in elderly men. *Aging Male*. 2002 Jun;5(2):98–102.

42. Cohen PG. Aromatase, adiposity, aging and disease. The hypogonadal-metabolic-atherogenic-disease and aging connection. Med Hypotheses. 2001 Jun;56(6):702–8.

43. Available at:http://www.acpinternist.org/archives/1999/11/epharm.htm. Accessed March 25, 2011.

44. Kent S. Crime report: Victory over the FDA. *Life Extension Magazine®*. 1996 Sept.

45. Zinman B, Harris SB, Neuman J, et al. Low-dose combination therapy with rosiglitazone and metformin to prevent type 2 diabetes mellitus (CANOE trial): a double-blind randomised controlled study. Lancet. 2010 Jul 10;376(9735):103–11.

46. Charles MA, Eschwege E. Prevention of type 2 diabetes: Role of Metformin. Drugs. 1999;58 Suppl.1:71–3; discussion 75–82.

47. Libby G, Donnelly LA, Donnan PT, Alessi DR, Morris AD, Evans JM. New users of metformin are at low risk of incident cancer: a cohort study among people with type 2 diabetes. Diabetes Care. 2009 Sep;32(9):1620–5.

48. Bodmer M, Meier C, Krahenbuhl S, Jick SS, Meier CR. Long-term metformin use is associated with decreased risk of breast cancer. Diabetes Care. 2010 Jun;33(6):1304–8.

49. Ben Sahra I, Laurent K, Giuliano S, et al. Targeting cancer cell metabolism: the combination of metformin and 2-deoxyglucose induces p53-dependent apoptosis in prostate cancer cells. Cancer Res. 2010 Mar 15;70(6):2465–75.

50. Rattan R, Giri S, Hartmann L, Shridhar V. Metformin attenuates ovarian cancer cell growth in an AMP-kinase dispensable manner. J Cell Mol Med. 2011 Jan;15(1):166–78.

51. Wang LW, Li ZS, Zou DW, Jin ZD, Gao J, Xu GM. Metformin induces apoptosis of pancreatic cancer cells. World J Gastroenterol. 2008 Dec 21;14(47):7192–8.

52. Memmott RM, Mercado JR, Maier CR, Kawabata S, Fox SD, Dennis PA. Metformin prevents tobacco carcinogen-induced lung tumorigenesis. Cancer Prev Res (Phila Pa). 2010 Sep;3(9):1066–76.

53. Algire C, Amrein L, Zakikhani M, Panasci L, Pollak M. Metformin blocks the stimulative effect of a high-energy diet on colon carcinoma growth in vivo and is associated with reduced expression of fatty acid synthase. Endocr Relat Cancer. 2010 Jun;17(2):351–60.

54. Stanosz S. An attempt at conservative treatment in selected cases of type I endometrial carcinoma (stage I a/G1) in young women. Eur J Gynaecol Oncol. 2009;30(4):365–9.

55. Faloon W. Consumer rape. *Life Extension Magazine*®. 2002 Apr.

56. Available at: http://www.cmpi.org/in-the-news/in-the-news/ growing-problem-of-fake-drugs-hurting-patients-companies/. Accessed March 25, 2011.

57. Bate R. Beware the Risks of Generic Drugs. *Wall Street Journal*. July 6, 2011.

58. Available at: http://www.fda.gov/NewsEvents/Newsroom/ PressAnnouncements/ucm242234.htm. Accessed March 25, 2011.

59. Available at: http://www.suntimes.com/lifestyles/health/ 4230222-423/company-hikes-preemie-preventive-drug-from-10-to-1500.html. Accessed March 28, 2011.

60. Available at: http://articles.latimes.com/2011/may/13/news/ la-pn-medicare-social-security-solvency-20110513. Accessed July 15, 2011.

61. Available at: http://voices.washingtonpost.com/federal-eye/2010/11/postal_service_posts_85_billio.html?nav=rss_ email/components. Accessed July 15, 2011.

Cancer: Is the "Standard of Care" the Best Treatment? Be Informed!

Cancer rates have either stabilized or increased, depending on the form of cancer, so that cancer is likely to become the leading cause of death in a few years. "Treatment" of cancer has become a gargantuan industry unto itself with cancer centers and cancer wings a must-have component of major hospitals. Billions of dollars are spent on cancer research, but no "cure" has been found, and it appears that only treatment offering billions of dollars of potential profit are welcome. This chapter explores the limitations of the current mainstream approach to cancer treatment and provides compelling evidence of some cutting-edge "unsanctioned" therapies that Life Extension® has pioneered. Anyone facing a cancer diagnoses should have this valuable information.

Assembly Line Medicine

PEOPLE FEAR CANCER more than any other disease—and for good reason. Upon diagnosis, a patient is often given several treatment choices. None guarantees a cure, but all tend to inflict pain, immobility, mutilation, debilitation, risk of secondary complications (like stroke), and risk of secondary cancers (like leukemia). Enlightened individuals face a particular degree of anxiety. They've heard about less toxic treatments that may be more effective. They often worry they are missing out on a curative therapy because of constraints placed on physicians by today's bureaucratic medical system that fosters inefficiency and mediocrity.

We at Life Extension® have long been aware of serious gaps that exist between what is discovered by cancer researchers and what is delivered to patients in the clinical oncology setting. When advanced cancer patients send us their medical records, we almost always identify treatment omissions that could have markedly improved odds of remission, improved survival, and even offered a cure. One example is a drug called cimetidine. It functions via several mechanisms to inhibit metastasis and improves survival in colon cancer patients.[1-8] In 2002, results from a clinical trial on patients with an aggressive form of colon cancer were published in the *British Journal of Cancer*. Compared to controls, 10-year survival improved by a remarkable 2.7-fold in the group receiving cimetidine.[4] Life Extension® has been recommending cimetidine since 1985 for certain types of cancer. Not once have we had a cancer patient approach us who had been prescribed this nontoxic drug by their oncologist.

An oncologist is a physician who specializes in the diagnosis, evaluation, and treatment of those afflicted with cancer. Cancer patients rely on their oncologist to utilize the best therapies to meet their individual needs. Regrettably, "managed care" has diluted the quality of care provided by many oncologists. In a stunning new development, a health insurance company is offering oncologists $350/month for each patient that is put on the company's recommended regimen.[9] This will enable the insurance company to control treatment-related expenses of cancer patients, who will be afforded less individualized, creative, and comprehensive care.

Within 24 hours of you reading this chapter, 1,500 Americans will perish from cancer.[10] There will be no sensational media accounts of these travesties, just more statistics to confirm the grim failure of mainstream medicine to find cures for this epidemic killer. We at Life Extension® have never ignored the threat that cancer poses to healthy longevity. Yet many people today are in a state of denial, as if this insidious disease only afflicts others. The news media redundantly covers details of traumatic deaths such as airline crashes and terrorist attacks. My reaction to these headline news stories is that the number of victims pales in comparison to the estimated 585,000 Americans that die from cancer every year.[11] As I wrote in a 2004 article titled "Are You Afraid of Terrorists?" over 2.4 million Americans die each year mostly from age-related disease. Yet one terrorist attack dominates media coverage.[12] So here we are 16 years later, and terrorists have killed less than 200 people in the United States. The death toll from cancer in that same time period is around 5.8 million. One could argue from a mathematical standpoint that violent death threats could be disregarded and resources instead poured into more efficient cancer research. My personal views don't directly relate to what you are about to read, but may help you understand how committed we are to eradicating cancer in the same way that smallpox was last century.

THE BASICS ABOUT CANCER TREATMENT

There are some basic rules about cancer that everyone should know. When it comes to achieving a "cure," the best opportunity exists at the time of first treatment. Once tumor cells have been exposed to initial therapies, or one's immune system has been compromised by surgical trauma, a malignancy can proliferate out of control and resist secondary therapeutic attempts.[13-20] The best shot for a cure thus involves an individualized, multipronged plan of action to:

- Eradicate the primary tumor;
- Decrease fuels that feed metastatic growth;
- Turn off stimuli that encourage cancer stem cell proliferation;
- Block the escape routes used by residual cancer cells.

Some people erroneously believe they must try to eradicate their tumor immediately. A more intelligent approach is to take the time needed to:

- Ensure that the stage or extent of the tumor is within the boundaries of any ablative therapy (such as surgery or radiation);

- Investigate every mechanism an individual's cancer will use to ensure its survival;
- Then introduce agents into the treatment protocol to circumvent each of these tumor survival factors.

What I'm conveying here is that newly diagnosed cancer patients should take advantage of the relatively vulnerable nature of their "treatment-naïve" tumor to implement a plan that addresses a wide range of escape routes that tumor cells utilize upon exposure to radiation, chemotherapy, hormone blockade, and even surgery.[21-25]

IMMUNE STATUS SHOULD BE ASSESSED IN ALL CANCER PATIENTS

Once a tumor is established, it is difficult for the immune system to eradicate it.[26-29] That's why mainstream oncologists pay little attention to the immune status of their newly diagnosed patients. In other words, since bolstering immune function alone won't cure cancer, oncologists mistakenly think it is not of major importance. Newly diagnosed patients often present with poor immune status even before immune-damaging chemotherapy, radiation, and/or surgery are initiated.[30-33]

Optimizing immune function prior to initiation of cancer treatment can be a critical component of comprehensive therapy with curative intent.[12,34-37] This involves in-depth immune profile blood testing and when indicated, precise administration of expensive drugs like interleukin-2,[12,38-46] filgrastim (Neupogen®),[47,48] pegfilgrastim (Neulasta®),[49-58] and/or sargramostim (Leukine®).[59-62] Health insurance companies are trying to reduce the cost of cancer care and would rather patients not know about the need to optimize immune function before, during, and after toxic therapies are administered.[63] The high cost of implementing comprehensive immune support is causing insurance companies to refuse to pay for it.

A large health insurance company is offering oncologists $350/month per patient as a reward to channel treatment toward the insurance company's "recommended regimen." We believe this will result in cancer patients dying sooner and using up fewer resources in the process.[8] Oncologists following these cookbook protocols will be able to squeeze far more patients into their hurried schedules. Under this new scheme whereby oncologists are paid $350/month for each patient placed on the "recommended regimen," insurance companies benefit financially, while patients are largely confined to chemo drug protocols that provide relatively minimal survival improvement in treating metastatic disease.

IMPACT OF SURGERY ON IMMUNE FUNCTION

The first line of defense against malignancy is our natural killer cells (NK). Young individuals have high levels of functional natural killer immune cells, but this declines with aging.[64–72] Natural killer cells originate in the bone marrow (like other immune cells) and go through a maturation process that enables them to participate in early control of microbial infections and cancers.[73–76] In a study examining NK cell activity in women shortly after surgery for breast cancer, it was reported that low levels of NK cell activity were associated with an increased risk of death from breast cancer.[77] In fact, reduced NK cell activity was a better predictor of survival than the actual stage of the cancer itself. In another study, colon cancer patients with reduced NK cell activity before surgery had a 350% increased risk of metastasis during the following 31 months.[78]

The likelihood of surgery-induced metastasis requires a cancer patient's immune system to be highly active and vigilant in seeking out and destroying renegade tumor cells immediately before, during, and after surgery. Numerous studies document that cancer surgery results in substantial reduction in NK cell activity.[79-82] In one investigation, NK cell activity in women having surgery for breast cancer was reduced by over 50% on the first day after surgery.[81] A group of researchers stated that, "We therefore believe that shortly after surgery, even transitory immune dysfunction might permit neoplasms [cancer] to enter the next stage of development and eventually form sizable metastases."[80]

We know cancer surgery reduces NK activity. This means that NK cell activity becomes impaired when it is most needed to fight metastasis. With that said, the preoperative and perioperative periods present a window of opportunity to actively strengthen immune function by enhancing NK cell activity. Fortunately, validated interventions to enhance NK cell activity are available to the person undergoing cancer surgery. While there are nutrients that can boost NK function, many cancer patients would benefit enormously with individualized courses of drugs like interleukin-2 (IL-2) and Leukine®. IL-2 directly promotes NK function,[83-85] while Leukine® induces bone marrow production of macrophages.[86-88] Since these drugs are expensive, insurance companies will often refuse to pay for them as they are not approved by the FDA for the creative interventions that published studies show may be effective.

HOW OFF-LABEL DRUGS SAVE LIVES

In the world of conventional oncology, FDA-approved drugs are routinely and legally prescribed for "unapproved uses" to better treat the disease.[89,90] This is often referred to as using drugs "off-label." A 2008 study found that eight out of 10 oncologists surveyed had used drugs off-label.[91] Studies have reported that about half of the chemotherapy drugs prescribed are for conditions not listed on the FDA-approved drug label.[92] The National Cancer Institute has stated, "Frequently the standard of care for a particular type or stage of cancer involves the off-label use of one or more drugs."[92] Off-label drug use in many cases is the genesis of innovation. It enables oncologists to use their training and experience to design creative therapeutic protocols based on new scientific findings. When favorable results are found, the protocol may be published in medical journals so that other oncologists can emulate the treatment successes.

The problem for health insurance companies is that cancer drugs are outlandishly priced, sometimes costing over $100,000 each per patient.[93–95] Insurance companies don't want to bear the costs associated with creatively designed treatments. They want to limit their expenses by confining oncologists to chemo drugs that provide relatively little survival improvement in advanced-stage cancers.[63] This helps explain why one insurance company is offering oncologists $350/month per patient to not prescribe drugs beyond the insurance company's "recommended regimen."[96] Other health insurance companies are doing it differently by reimbursing oncologists less money when they prescribe newer, more expensive cancer drugs.[97]

NOT ALL OFF-LABEL DRUGS ARE EXPENSIVE

Some of the most effective off-label drugs are affordable out-of-pocket (without insurance company involvement). The problem occurs when oncologists are being paid ($350/month) to only offer an insurance company's "recommended regimen." This creates a disincentive to utilize Herculean initiatives to ensure their patients receive every therapy that could optimize outcomes with the goal of inducing a complete remission; in other words, the complete disappearance of all manifestations of the cancer.

From our review of the scientific literature spanning decades, many cancer patients would benefit by taking aspirin[98–100] and the antidiabetic drug metformin.[101–115] Aspirin of course is readily accessible, but cancer patients are unlikely to use it if their oncologist does not recommend it. Metformin requires a prescription, and if the insurance company catches the oncologist prescribing metformin, which is not part of the "recommended regimen," the oncologist might lose the $350/month stipend for that patient. Even the use of aspirin requires the oncologist's involvement as chemo patients whose platelet count is reduced to fewer than $100 \times 10E^3/uL$ are at risk for hemorrhage.[116–119] Under these circumstances, aspirin should be deferred until platelet counts are restored.

There are numerous off-label drugs effective against certain cancers (such as COX-2 inhibitors, certain statins, hormone modulators, etc.) that require a prescription, yet we are rapidly regressing to a system where medical decision-making is dictated by insurance company cost mandates and not physician dedication and experience.

HOW POSITIVE RESPONSES TO CANCER THERAPY ARE DEFINED

- **Partial remission (PR)** indicates 50% or greater reduction in all measureable evidence of tumor dimensions and tumor markers.
- **Complete remission (CR)** indicates a disappearance of all measureable indicators of tumor activity.
- **Cure** indicates complete disappearance of all manifestations of disease activity that is sustained over years and insures a high probability that the disease will not return.

Cancer patients can derive survival benefits when adjuvant therapies are combined with conventional treatments.

THE INSURANCE COMPANY'S "RECOMMENDED REGIMEN"

The chemotherapy drugs that insurance companies want oncologists to prescribe represent the most commonly used drugs in the industry and can be viewed as aggressive "cookbook medicine approach" treatments. Some of drugs listed, such as Adriamycin®, are being limited by several oncologists at major medical institutions, such as M. D. Anderson, for use in adjuvant settings due to excessive toxicity.[121–123] Progressive oncologists, with whom Life Extension® is working, are using mitoxantrone instead of Adriamycin® in their elderly patients since it has the same survival rate as Adriamycin®, but is less toxic to the heart.[124–126]

Oncologists will be paid $350/month per patient by one insurer to prescribe chemo drugs such as Adriamycin®, which was approved by the FDA in 1974. Another insurer is offering higher reimbursement to the oncologist when lower-cost chemo drugs are used. All these chemo drugs are considered standard of care by the National Comprehensive Cancer Network, which is an alliance of 25 cancer centers in the United States, most of which are designated by the National Cancer Institute as comprehensive cancer centers. Health insurance companies reward practicing oncologists for following the standard published protocols that minimize creative approaches for cancer treatment.

Perhaps the greatest failing of the chemo drugs that insurers are paying oncologists to prescribe is that they seldom cure advanced-stage cancers. Despite widespread availability of these chemo drugs, metastatic lung cancer kills 98% of patients within five years.[127] Metastatic colon cancer kills 94% within five years.[128] Those afflicted with metastatic breast cancer fare better, but 78% still die within five years.[129]

Clinical oncology practice clearly needs more innovation—yet health insurance companies are providing financial incentives for physicians to prescribe chemo drugs that fail to cure advanced-stage patients. This kind of backwards approach to treatment will stifle the discovery of breakthroughs so desperately needed to spare the lives of more than 585,000 Americans who perish from cancer annually. I'm purposely leaving the names of the insurance companies out of this chapter because it is likely that other insurers will follow this pattern of scientific regression. What we are witnessing is clinical oncology practice being driven backward by outlandish drug prices, along with the high cost of increased physician involvement when aggressive therapies are utilized. Health insurance companies argue their "recommended regimens" will improve patient care. We at Life Extension® disagree and advocate that more (not fewer) individualized, creative, and comprehensive treatment approaches could spare numerous lives.

THE PROBLEM WITH CYTOTOXIC (CHEMOTHERAPY) DRUGS

When chemotherapy drugs were developed in the 1950s to 1970s, there was optimism that a pharmaceutical cure for cancer might soon be found. These chemo drugs killed cancer cells in the petri dish and shrank tumors in cancer patients. The side effects, however, were horrific, and survival improvements were negligible for most solid malignancies. Medical oncologists are now being offered $350/month per patient to prescribe chemo drugs that, in some cases, were introduced before many of you reading this chapter were born. There are drugs in the insurance company's "recommended regimen" that are new and considered cutting-edge, but provide average survival improvements often measuring less than one year.

In the May 21, 2014 edition of the *Journal of the American Medical Association*, a study was published showing that lung cancer patients survived 1.1 years longer when aggressive genomic testing was done and drugs that specifically target an individual tumor are added to standard chemo regimens.[120] These newer drugs target what's known as "oncogenic drivers," which are genetic abnormalities critical for tumor development and maintenance. The survival improvement in response to these "targeted" therapies is certainly welcomed news, but a far cry from a cure. The side effects from these newer cancer drugs are similar to old-line chemo drugs, meaning the patients endure significant suffering in exchange for added time.

Our scientific understanding of molecular oncology has grown exponentially over the past 40 to 50 years, yet relatively little of this knowledge is being delivered to the cancer patient. Clinical oncology practice, in fact, has progressed so slowly that many old-line chemo drugs are still considered first-line therapy at cancer institutions today, despite their failures to produce cures in the majority of advanced cases.

The problem is that consumers with health insurance may not have a choice. If their oncologist follows the insurers "recommended regimen," they will be prescribed chemo drugs that have historically provided relatively minimal survival improvement. These patients might better benefit from creative therapies that health insurance companies now balk at paying for.

The columns on the next page list chemotherapy drugs that one insurance company wants most of its insured customers restricted to, along with the dates of each drug's approval and how many years each of these drugs has been in use. Some of these drugs were approved more than 60 years ago. That does not mean they are not still useful against certain malignancies. The invariable question is whether certain patients who would benefit from more comprehensive and creative approaches will instead be prescribed these "standard-of-care" drugs because of the financial incentives being offered to oncologists. To receive their $350/month stipend per patient, oncologists have to stay with the insurance company's "recommended regimen" for that patient. This financial incentive comes to $4,200 a year per patient treated following the insurer's protocol!

Drug Name	Approval Date	Years In Use
Leucovorin	June 20, 1952	62
Cyclophosphamide (Cytoxan®)	November 16, 1959 (Manufacturing changes in 1976, 1977, 1979, 1984, 1987, 2000 Cytoxan® (lyophilized) equivalent	55
Fluorouracil (5-FU)	April 25, 1962	52
DoxorubicinHCL injectable (Adriamycin®)	August 7, 1974	39
Cisplatin (Platinol®)	December 19, 1978	35
Carboplatin (Paraplatin®)	March 3, 1989	25
Paclitaxel (Taxol®)	December 29, 1992 (Manufacturing change or addition 1993, 1994, 1997, 1998, 2001)	21
Vinorelbine (Navelbine®)	December 23, 1994	19
Docetaxel (Taxotere®)	May 14, 1996	18
Gemcitabine (Gemzar®)	May 15, 1996	18
Irinotecan (Camptosar®)	June 14, 1996	18
Capecitabine (Xeloda®)	April 30, 1998	16
Trastuzumab (Herceptin®)	September 25, 1998 (Manufacturing change 2012)	15

Drug Name	Approval Date	Years In Use
Epirubicin (Ellence®)	September 15, 1999	14
Oxaliplatin (Eloxatin®)	August 9, 2002	11
Pemetrexed (Alimta®)	February 4, 2004	10
Bevacizumab (Avastin®)	February 26, 2004	10
Erlotinib (Tarceva®)	November 18, 2004	9
Panitumumab (Vectibix®)	September 27, 2006	7
Lapatinib(Tykerb®)	March 13, 2007	7
Pertuzumab (Perjeta®)	June 8, 2012	2
Regorafenib (Stivarga®)	September 27, 2012	1
Ado-trastuzumabemtansine (Kadcyla®)	February 22, 2013	1
Afatinib (Gilotrif®)	July 12, 2013	1
Average age of chemo drug		19

MOST EFFECTIVE BRAIN TUMOR DRUG NOT APPROVED TO TREAT ANY CANCER

Perhaps the most frightening malignancy one can be diagnosed with is a form of brain cancer called glioblastoma. This type of brain cancer has a dismal prognosis, with median overall survival of 12 to 14 months, and a two-year survival rate of 15 to 26%.[131] Senator Ted Kennedy was diagnosed with glioblastoma in May 2008. Despite intervention by some of the best brain tumor experts, Kennedy died in August 2009—a mere 15 months later. A study published in the *New England Journal of Medicine* on September 5, 2013, may represent the most significant advance yet discovered in treating glioblastoma.[131]What follows is an overview of a drug that is not approved to treat any cancer, and thus is likely to be rejected by insurance company mandates:

- Valganciclovir (Valcyte®) is an FDA-approved drug used to treat cytomegalovirus infection.
- Cytomegalovirus has been suspected as facilitating the initiation and promotion of brain cancers.[132–135] Some 50 to 80% of adults in the US show exposure to cytomegalovirus, but relatively few harbor active viral infection.[135]
- Doctors followed 75 glioblastoma patients and found the median overall survival of those with low-grade cytomegalovirus infection was 33 months. In patients with high-grade cytomegalovirus infection, median overall survival was 13 months.[131]
- All but one of the 75 glioblastoma patients studied had active cytomegalovirus infection, indicating that this virus may be involved in the development of this lethal malignancy. [131]
- In glioblastoma patients with high-grade cytomegalovirus infection, median two-year survival was 17.2%. Patients with low-grade cytomegalovirus infection had median two-year survival rates of 63.6%.[131] This suggests that high-grade, active cytomegalovirus infection accelerates tumor progression.
- In a double-blind clinical trial of valganciclovir involving 42 patients with glioblastoma, an exploratory analysis of 22 patients receiving at least six months of antiviral therapy showed 50% overall survival at two years compared with 20.6% of contemporary controls.[131] This study showed that valganciclovir-treated patients had a median overall survival of 24.1 months

compared to 13.7 months in patients not treated with valganciclovir.

- Owing to the promising results of this pilot study, physicians at the world-famous Karolinska University Hospital administered valganciclovir to glioblastoma patients, and results were then compared to a control group. Both groups received standard conventional therapy and both groups had a similar disease stage and surgical-resection grade.

- The researchers retrospectively analyzed the data on 50 of these brain cancer patients and found the two-year rate of survival in the valganciclovir group was 62%, whereas two-year survival was only 18% in the control group.[131]

- In 40 glioblastoma patients who received valganciclovir for at least six months, the two-year survival rate was 70%, with a median overall survival of 30.1 months.[131]

- In 25 glioblastoma patients who received continuous valganciclovir treatment after the first six months, the two-year survival rate was 90%, with a median overall survival of 56.4 months (4.7 years)![131]

- The current median survival of glioblastoma patients is only 12 to 14 months (1.0 to 1.16 years).[131] The efforts made to prolong Senator Kennedy's life by the experts at Duke University Medical Center was a survival of 15 months (1.25 years)—3.45 years less than the median survival in the 25 glioblastoma patients who received continuous valganciclovir treatment as detailed above.

The implication from these findings is that treating active cytomegalovirus infection may dramatically reduce progression, and significantly increase survival time, in

patients suffering from the deadly brain cancer glioblastoma. Most exciting is the intriguing data from this retrospective study showing that in glioblastoma patients with
active cytomegalovirus, a treatment protocol employing
valganciclovir resulted in a median survival of 4.7 years!
Not only does this retrospective data involving the continuous use of valganciclovir substantially extend survival in
glioblastoma patients, but it also provides an opportunity
to incorporate additional complementary therapies that
could improve survival even more!

WHY BRAIN TUMOR PATIENTS ARE DENIED VALGANCICLOVIR

It is illegal for the maker of valganciclovir to promote it
as a treatment for brain cancer. The regulatory system
in the United States requires that the maker of a drug
conduct extensive clinical trials for each disease a drug
claims to treat and then submit the trial results to the
FDA for approval. It is not illegal, however, for an oncologist to prescribe valganciclovir to treat glioblastoma. The
problem is the annual cost for valganciclovir is around
$50,000. Many health insurers will refuse to pay this out-
landish price. If an oncologist tries to prescribe it for a
patient it will not be one of the insurance company's "recommended regimens," and the oncologists will likely lose
his $350/month stipend because he or she did not adhere
to the treatment protocols designated by the insurer. We
fear that 12,000 Americans will continue to die prematurely from glioblastoma every year despite impressive
findings showing that valganciclovir could extend the
survival times of many of these patients diagnosed with
this deadly disease.[136]

**INDUSTRY ACTUARIES GUIDE
YOUR CANCER TREATMENT**

The practice of medicine has largely devolved to a place where physicians no longer take the lead in guiding treatment. Consider a scenario that plays out day after day in modern cancer treatment. An experienced oncologist sees a Medicare patient suffering from an aggressive cancer. The oncologist realizes that there are several viable options, and that the best therapy is not the usual, cost-effective standard-of-care choice covered by Medicare. Rather, it's a more expensive and newer option with compelling data that shows better results. However, the newer, more expensive treatment option—the one that's best for the patient in the opinion of the treating oncologist—is not standard of care and therefore, is not covered under Medicare.

The result? The patient is treated with the Medicare-approved drug. In this case, the federal government's actuaries at the Center for Medicare & Medicaid Services have been the guiding force in treatment of this patient, not the experienced oncologist.

CHANGING CANCER CARE FOR THE WORSE

What we are seeing before our eyes are physicians who will give up years of education, creativity, and understanding of the individual patient to instead be directed by an insurance company and rewarded with a monthly stipend of $350 if he or she follows the insurers financially biased "orders." The term now used for physicians in such a context is "provider." They provide the treatment, but are not involved in deciding what treatments to use. Thus, the physician has given up his or her role as "Decider" to become the "Provider."

The $350/month per patient could possibly be a significant income for the oncologist. Assume that oncologist has 400 active patients and that 100 of them are on the insurers "approved" chemo program. That's $35,000 per month or $420,000 per year. In most major cities, that's about what the average medical oncologist makes annually. If the oncologist surrenders his decision-making to the insurer, he is doing less work and has fewer worries regarding patient outcome since he was only "following orders." The insurance company decided on the regimen. Thus, the trade-off to surrender physician autonomy for a substantial monetary reward that involves less stress on the physician becomes an irresistible temptation for far too many highly educated and highly trained medical oncologists.

Another concern is what will the insurer decide regarding the use of supportive care therapy, such as antiemetic and immune protective treatment prior to chemo. What will the insurer mandate regarding which imaging studies can or cannot be done, what laboratory studies are to be obtained and how often, and which immune-augmenting drugs are to be used? Where does the direction of care involving cost-cutting stop? In this newly perverse system brought about by outlandishly high medical prices, why bother using physicians to treat cancer patients? Given this form of cookbook medicine, costs could be further cut by using nurse practitioners or physician assistants to deliver standard care chemo drugs.

> Insurers are changing how they pay for cancer care, aiming to blunt soaring costs and push oncologists to adhere to standardized treatment guidelines.[130]
>
> *Wall Street Journal*, May 27, 2014

BLAME THE BROKEN SYSTEM . . . NOT JUST INSURANCE COMPANIES

A number of health insurance companies are looking into aggressive ways to cut the soaring costs of cancer drugs by seeking to reduce payments to oncologists if they prescribe pricier drugs. Of the 12 new cancer drugs approved in 2012, 11 were priced above $100,000 a year! Over a hundred oncologists signed a protest letter that concluded that the prices of many of these drugs "are too high, unsustainable, may compromise access of needy patients to highly effective therapy, and are harmful to the sustainability of our national healthcare systems."[137]

Now we are seeing insurance companies rebel by offering incentives to oncologists to prescribe chemo drugs they perceive as being less expensive. Here is a quote from the insurance company's oncology medical director:[138]

> This program—while sharing best practices and evidence-based medicine—also helps to support oncologists who require large staffs to treat these complex patients and provides the practice with enhanced reimbursement to offset the lower fees they receive when prescribing less expensive drugs.

According to the IMS Institute for Healthcare Informatics, in 2013 the United States spent $37 billion on cancer drugs, which is more than any other category.[139] Overall costs for treating cancer are well over $100 billion annually and mounting steadily, according to researchers at the National Cancer Institute. Hospital, diagnostic, and pharmaceutical prices are beyond exorbitant.

A patient under the guidance of the International Strategic Cancer Alliance (ISCA) was recently charged $2,500 for a bone density outpatient test at a prestigious university hospital.

The going rate at a diagnostic testing center is around $250. When ISCA responded by threatening to pay for an advertisement in the *New York Times* indicating this abuse by the university hospital, the hospital drastically reduced their price to this patient (but not to other cash-paying patients).

Still another reason why medical costs are spiraling upward is large hospitals that are buying out individual oncology practices so higher "hospital" prices can be billed to Medicare, Medicaid, and health insurance companies. When chemo is administered in an oncologist's private office, the cost is less than compared to a hospital setting. Now hospitals are employing oncologists to make sure patients receive chemo in the hospital's oncology outpatient facility and billing insurance company's higher prices, which means you will be paying higher health insurance premiums, along with higher co-pays and deductibles.

The financial coffers of insurance companies are being plundered by the excess charges of hospitals and outrageously high drug prices. Insurance companies are responding by seeking to pay doctors to provide less costly treatments. This is bad news for cancer victims. It is important to point out that in many clinical oncology settings, the insurance company's new "recommended regimens" may not be any worse than what patients are getting anyway. Bureaucracies have replaced the "special" physician, the one that comes up with creative approaches and who devours the literature looking for clues to help save his or her patient. Mainstream mediocrity has become the "standard of care" in too many instances, and the public apathetically accepts it until they or a loved one is stricken with cancer.

The major factor responsible for the decay and dysfunction of sick-care in the US is the powerful pharmaceutical lobby, the health insurance industry, and the burdensome legislation enacted by Congress that stifles innovation in the medical arena. None of these revelations should surprise Life Extension® followers, who long ago learned how regulatory strangleholds inflict harsh economic pain, along with needless suffering and death.

AGGRESSIVE APPROACHES CAN CURE TERMINAL CANCER

In April of 2000, a patient came to us with advanced head and neck cancer with a primary location in the sinus and infiltration to the brain and orbital (eye) cavity. The tumor was the approximate size of a baseball and every oncologist consulted stated the patient had only months to live. Hospice was recommended as there was no conventional therapy that could treat this patient due to the complex anatomical locations of the tumor.

Just imagine the challenge of treating a tumor of this size growing inside someone's head. The tumor's location made it untreatable, according to every oncology expert. The only advantage we had is that no treatment had yet been administered, meaning the tumor was "treatment naïve," and thus vulnerable to eradication by multimodal therapies. Our dilemma was figuring out how to administer therapy to this delicate anatomical region of the body without blinding the patient and creating permanent brain damage. The hospital wanted to administer systemic cisplatin chemotherapy, which would have temporarily shrunk the tumor, but at the cost of horrific side effects and the mutation of the tumor to a virtually invulnerable stage. We stopped the patient from getting the systemic cisplatin in the nick of time.

The scientific team at Life Extension® devised an unprecedented protocol that involved inserting a catheter into the patient's femoral artery. The catheter was directed into the aorta and from there threaded into the external carotid arteries. Using the catheter as a chemotherapy delivery system to the tumor, a relatively massive dose of cisplatin was initially used to target the tumor. It would have been impossible to deliver enough of this highly toxic chemo drug in any other way. Even by delivering cisplatin directly into the tumor, there were still some side effects (renal impairment) which were able to be reversed. Following initial direct-to-the-tumor cisplatin therapy, the chemo drug paclitaxel was administered via this same intra-arterial route for four additional weeks.

These intra-arterial chemotherapy sessions were immediately followed by proton beam-accelerated radiation and the use of numerous drugs not approved to treat this cancer. For example, to enhance the tumor-killing effects of the proton beam-accelerated radiation, the radiation sensitizer 3-chloroprocainamide (3-CPA) was used. This had to be synthesized in our lab, as it was not commercially available to us. To further enhance the proton-beam therapy, the patient ingested 18 grams of arginine before treatment and breathed pure oxygen during treatment. The objective was to thoroughly oxygenate the patient in order to induce maximal tumor cell death during the proton-beam therapy.

It took until late June 2000 (the patient was diagnosed in April 2000) to initiate this complex therapy. By September 2000, there was no sign of active tumor. The patient was in complete remission, meaning there was no sign of tumor activity in the patient's body. Oncologists at Loma Linda Medical Center were so impressed that they used this same protocol on another patient with advanced sinus cancer. We were informed that in this patient a complete remission was also attained.

Our client was prescribed a three-year follow up cyclical dosing of interferon alfa-2b and 13-cis retinoic acid to mop up any residual tumor cells that may have escaped the aggressive proton beam and intra-arterial chemo that was delivered over an eight-week time period. Within two years, our client developed radiation necrosis of the brain, which was caused by the high dose of proton beam radiation therapy. This is a common side effect when the brain is irradiated. Once again, conventional doctors pronounced our client "terminal," since there was no recognized treatment to overcome the raging inflammatory fires destroying the brain.

The scientific team here at Life Extension® went back to work and identified two drugs (cabergoline and pentoxifylline), both not approved to treat radiation necrosis. The two-drug combination suppressed the radiation necrosis, and once again to the doctor's amazement, this patient was cured of a side effect that had been pronounced terminal. Our client remains alive today, 14 years since the original "terminal" diagnosis was made. To make more of these kinds of lifesaving therapies available, I helped set up the International Strategic Cancer Alliance (ISCA) to speed innovative cancer treatments to patients who are unable to be helped by conventional oncology.

WHAT WE ARE DOING TO SAVE LIVES

For over 37 years, we at Life Extension® have relentlessly combatted the high cost of medicine, along with conventional oncology's less-than-optimal approach to cancer treatment. We offer two services for our supporters who develop cancer. One is free phone/email access to our cancer advisors. There is seldom a call where we can't suggest validated ways to improve survival, sometimes as simple as adding aspirin and metformin to conventional treatment. To speak with a cancer advisor, call 1-866-864-3027.

The second option is concierge oversight provided by the International Strategic Cancer Alliance (ISCA). This service has collectively lost us millions of dollars since its inception, but in the process has saved lives and added life-years. The main cost when using the International Strategic Cancer Alliance has been the high hourly rates charged by top-notch oncologists and other personnel involved in developing personalized and creative treatment strategies. New health insurance exclusions may also increase the patient's out-of-pocket costs when utilizing ISCA's Personalized Treatment Protocols. To reach out to the International Strategic Cancer Alliance, call 1-610-628-3419.

QUOTE FROM AYN RAND REGARDING DOCTORS

I have often wondered at the smugness with which people assert their right to enslave me, to control my work, to force my will, to violate my conscience, to stifle my mind, yet what is it that they expect to depend on, when they lie on an operating table under my hands? Let them discover the kind of doctors that their system will now produce. Let them discover, in their operating rooms and hospital wards that it is not safe to place their lives in the hands of a man whose life they have throttled. It is not safe, if he is the sort of man who resents it—and still less safe, if he is the sort who doesn't.

—*Atlas Shrugged,* Ayn Rand

References

1. Lefranc F, Yeaton P, Brotchi J, Kiss R. Cimetidine, an unexpected anti-tumor agent, and its potential for the treatment of glioblastoma. *Int J Oncol.* 2006 May;28(5):1021–30.

2. Natori T, Sata M, Nagai R, Makuuchi M. Cimetidine inhibits angiogenesis and suppresses tumor growth. *Biomed Pharmacother.* 2005 Jan-Feb;59(1–2):56–60.

3. Tomita K, Izumi K, Okabe S. Roxatidine-and cimetidine-induced angiogenesis inhibition suppresses growth of colon cancer implants in syngeneic mice. *J Pharmacol Sci.* 2003 Nov;93(3):321–30.

4. Matsumoto S, Imaeda Y, Umemoto S, Kobayashi K, Suzuki H, Okamoto T. Cimetidine increases survival of colorectal cancer patients with high levels of sialyl Lewis-X and sialyl

Lewis-A epitope expression on tumour cells. *Br J Cancer.* 2002 Jan 21;86(2):161–7.

5. Adams WJ, Lawson JA, Morris DL. Cimetidine inhibits in vivo growth of human colon cancer and reverses histamine stimulated in vitro and in vivo growth. *Gut.* 1994 Nov;35(11):1632–6.

6. Adams WJ, Lawson JA, Nicholson SE, Cook TA, Morris DL. The growth of carcinogen-induced colon cancer in rats is inhibited by cimetidine. *Eur J Surg Oncol.* 1993 Aug;19 (4):332–5.

7. Adams WJ, Morris DL, Ross WB, Lubowski DZ, King DW, Peters L. Cimetidine preserves nonspecific immune function after colonic resection for cancer. *Aust N Z J Surg.* 1994 Dec;64(12):847–52.

8. Adams WJ, Morris DL. Short-course cimetidine and survival with colorectal cancer. *Lancet.* 1994 Dec 24–31;344 (8939–8940):1768–9.

9. Available at: http://webreprints.djreprints.com/34053314 20659.html. Accessed June 24, 2014.

10. Available at:http://www.forecancerresearch.org/cancerfacts. aspx. Accessed July 12, 2014.

11. Available at: http://seer.cancer.gov/statfacts/html/all.html. Accessed July 12, 2014.

12. Available at: http://www.lef.org/magazine/mag2004/jun2004_ awsi_01.htm. Accessed July 12, 2014.

13. Brivio F, Lissoni P, Rovelli F, et al. Effects of IL-2 preoperative immunotherapy on surgery-induced changes in angiogenic regulation and its prevention of VEGF increase and IL-12 decline. *Hepatogastroenterology.* 2002 Mar-Apr;49(44):385–7.

14. Shankaran V, Ikeda H, Bruce AT, et al. IFN gamma and lymphocytes prevent primary tumour development and shape tumour immunogenicity. *Nature.* 2001 Apr 26;410(6832):1107–11.

15. Fadul CE, Fisher JL, Hampton TH, et al. Immune response in patients with newly diagnosed glioblastoma multiforme

treated with intranodal autologous tumor lysate-dendritic cell vaccination after radiation chemotherapy. *J Immunother.* 2011 May;34(4):382–9.

16. Seeger RC. Immunology and immunotherapy of neuroblastoma. *Semin Cancer Biol.* 2011 Oct;21(4):229–37.

17. Louis CU, Savoldo B, Dotti G, et al. Antitumor activity and long-term fate of chimeric antigen receptor-positive T cells in patients with neuroblastoma. *Blood.* 2011 Dec 1;118(23):6050–6.

18. Ardon H, Van Gool S, Lopes IS, et al. Integration of autologous dendritic cell-based immunotherapy in the primary treatment for patients with newly diagnosed glioblastoma multiforme: a pilot study. *J Neurooncol.* 2010 Sep;99(2):261–72.

19. Smith C, Tsang J, Beagley L, et al. Effective treatment of metastatic forms of Epstein-Barr virus-associated nasopharyngeal carcinoma with a novel adenovirus-based adoptive immunotherapy. *Cancer Res.* 2012 Mar 1;72(5):1116–25.

20. Miles SA, Sandler AD. CpG oligonucleotides for immunotherapeutic treatment of neuroblastoma. *Adv Drug Deliv Rev.* 2009 Mar 28;61(3):275–82.

21. Available at: http://www.newscientist.com/article/dn21516-new-cancer-drug-sabotages-tumours-escape-route.html#.U9KXM3l0yUk. Accessed June 25, 2014.

22. Available at: http://www.sciencedaily.com/releases/2013/02/130226135525.htm. Accessed June 25, 2014.

23. Hoogstraat M, de Pagter MS, Cirkel GA, van Roosmalen M J, Harkins TT, Duran, K, et al. Genomic and transcriptomic plasticity in treatment-naïve ovarian cancer. *Genome Res.* 2014 Feb;24(2):200–11.

24. Attar RM, Takimoto CH, Gottardis MM. Castration-resistant prostate cancer: locking up the molecular escape routes. *Clin Cancer Res.* 2009;15(10):3251–55.

25. Available at: http://www.newscientist.com/article/mg22029441.700-beating-cancer-by-blocking-off-its-escape-routes.html#.U8PtvnlOWUk. Accessed July 14, 2014.

26. Huang Y, Shah S, Qiao L. Tumor resistance to CD8+ T cell-based therapeutic vaccination. *Arch Immunol Ther Exp (Warsz)*. 2007 Jul-Aug;55(4):205–17.

27. Huang Y, Obholzer N, Fayad R, Qiao L. Turning on/off tumor-specific CTL response during progressive tumor growth. *J Immunol*. 2005 Sep 1;175(5):3110–6.

28. Speiser DE, Ohashi PS. Activation of cytotoxic T cells by solid tumours? *Cell Mol Life Sci*. 1998 Mar;54(3):263–71.

29. Igney FH, Krammer PH. Immune escape of tumors: apoptosis resistance and tumor counterattack. *J Leukoc Biol*. 2002 Jun;71(6):907–20.

30. Sun S, Fei X, Mao Y, et al. PD-1(+) immune cell infiltration inversely correlates with survival of operable breast cancer patients. *Cancer Immunol Immunother*. 2014 Apr;63(4):395–406.

31. Huang JJ, Jiang WQ, Lin TY, et al. Absolute lymphocyte count is a novel prognostic indicator in extranodal natural killer/T-cell lymphoma, nasal type. *Ann Oncol*. 2011 Jan;22(1):149–55.

32. Xu L, Xu W, Qiu S, Xiong S. Enrichment of CCR6+Foxp3+ regulatory T cells in the tumor mass correlates with impaired CD8+ T cell function and poor prognosis of breast cancer. *Clin Immunol*. 2010 Jun;135(3):466–75.

33. Masmoudi A, Toumi N, Khanfir A, et al. Epstein-Barr virus-targeted immunotherapy for nasopharyngeal carcinoma. *Cancer Treat Rev*. 2007 Oct;33(6):499–505.

34. Angelini C, Bovo G, Muselli P, et al. Preoperative interleukin-2 immunotherapy in pancreatic cancer: preliminary results. *Hepatogastroenterology*. 2006 Jan-Feb;53(67):141–4.

35. Ratto GB, Costa R, Maineri P, et al. Neo-adjuvant chemo/immunotherapy in the treatment of stage III (N2) non-small cell lung cancer: a phase I/II pilot study. *Int J Immunopathol Pharmacol*. 2011 Oct-Dec;24(4):1005–16.

36. Ludgate CM. Optimizing cancer treatments to induce an acute immune response: radiation Abscopal effects, PAMPs, and DAMPs. *Clin Cancer Res*. 2012 Sep 1;18(17):4522–5.

37. Sarkar S, Döring A, Zemp FJ, et al. Therapeutic activation of macrophages and microglia to suppress brain tumor-initiating cells. *Nat Neurosci.* 2014 Jan;17(1):46–55.

38. Antony GK, Dudek AZ. Interleukin 2 in cancer therapy. *Curr Med Chem.* 2010;17(29):3297–302.

39. Maroto JP, del Muro XG, Mellado B, et al. Phase II trial of sequential subcutaneous interleukin-2 plus interferon alpha followed by sorafenib in renal cell carcinoma (RCC). *Clin Transl Oncol.* 2013 Sep;15(9):698–704.

40. Weide B, Eigentler TK, Pflugfelder A, et al. Survival after intratumoral interleukin-2 treatment of 72 melanoma patients and response upon the first chemotherapy during follow-up. *Cancer Immunol Immunother.* 2011 Apr;60(4):487–93.

41. Slavin S, Ackerstein A, Or R, et al. Immunotherapy in high-risk chemotherapy-resistant patients with metastatic solid tumors and hematological malignancies using intentionally mismatched donor lymphocytes activated with rIL-2: a phase I study. *Cancer Immunol Immunother.* 2010 Oct;59(10):1511–9.

42. Vuoristo MS, Vihinen P, Skyttä T, Tyynelä K, Kellokumpu-Lehtinen P. Carboplatin and vinorelbine combined with subcutaneous interleukin-2 in metastatic melanoma with poor prognosis. *Anticancer Res.* 2009 May;29(5):1755–9.

43. Hallett WH, Ames E, Alvarez M, et al. Combination therapy using IL-2 and anti-CD25 results in augmented natural killer cell-mediated antitumor responses. *Biol Blood Marrow Transplant.* 2008 Oct;14(10):1088–99.

44. Lissoni P, Brivio F, Fumagalli L, Di Fede G, Brera G. Enhancement of the efficacy of chemotherapy with oxaliplatin plus 5-fluorouracil by pretreatment with IL-2 subcutaneous immunotherapy in metastatic colorectal cancer patients with lymphocytopenia prior to therapy. *In Vivo.* 2005 Nov-Dec;19(6):1077–80.

45. Quan WD Jr, Quan FM, Perez M, Johnson E. Outpatient intravenous interleukin-2 with famotidine has activity in metastatic melanoma. *Cancer Biother Radiopharm*. 2012 Sep;27(7):442–5.

46. Hanzly M, Aboumohamed A, Yarlagadda N, et al. High-dose interleukin-2 therapy for metastatic renal cell carcinoma: a contemporary experience. *Urology*. 2014 May;83(5):1129–34.

47. Schäfer H, Hübel K, Bohlen H, et al. Perioperative treatment with filgrastim stimulates granulocyte function and reduces infectious complications after esophagectomy. *Ann Hematol*. 2000 Mar;79(3):143–51.

48. Wenisch C, Werkgartner T, Sailer H, et al. Effect of preoperative prophylaxis with filgrastim in cancer neck dissection. *Eur J Clin Invest*. 2000 May;30(5):460–6.

49. Hill G, Barron R, Fust K, et al. Primary vs secondary prophylaxis with pegfilgrastim for the reduction of febrile neutropenia risk in patients receiving chemotherapy for non-Hodgkin's lymphoma: cost-effectiveness analyses. *J Med Econ*. 2014 Jan;17(1):32–42.

50. Tesařová P. OPERa Study. *Klin Onkol (Czech)*. 2013 26(6):425–33.

51. Naeim A, Henk HJ, Becker L, Chia V, Badre S, Li X, Deeter R. Pegfilgrastim prophylaxis is associated with a lower risk of hospitalization of cancer patients than filgrastim prophylaxis: a retrospective United States claims analysis of granulocyte colony-stimulating factors (G-CSF). *BMC Cancer*. 2013 Jan 8;13:11.

52. Hadji P, Kostev K, Schröder-Bernhardi D, Ziller V. Cost comparison of outpatient treatment with granulocyte colony-stimulating factors (G-CSF) in Germany. *Int J Clin Pharmacol Ther*. 2012 Apr;50(4):281–9.

53. Hirsch BR, Lyman GH. Pharmacoeconomics of the myeloid growth factors: a critical and systematic review. *Pharmacoeconomics*. 2012 Jun 1;30(6):497–511.

54. Aapro MS, Bohlius J, Cameron DA, et al. European Organisation for Research and Treatment of Cancer. 2010 update of EORTC guidelines for the use of granulocyte-colony stimulating factor to reduce the incidence of chemotherapy-induced febrile neutropenia in adult patients with lymphoproliferative disorders and solid tumours. *Eur J Cancer*. 2011 Jan;47(1):8–32.

55. Bonanno G, Procoli A, Mariotti A, et al. Effects of pegylated G-CSF on immune cell number and function in patients with gynecological malignancies. *J Transl Med*. 2010 Nov 9;8:114.

56. Sehouli J, Goertz A, Steinle T, et al. Pegfilgrastim vs filgrastim in primary prophylaxis of febrile neutropenia in patients with breast cancer after chemotherapy: a cost-effectiveness analysis for Germany. *Dtsch Med Wochenschr*. 2010 Mar;135(9):385–9.

57. Lyman G, Lalla A, Barron R, Dubois RW. Cost-effectiveness of pegfilgrastim versus 6-day filgrastim primary prophylaxis in patients with non-Hodgkin's lymphoma receiving CHOP-21 in United States. *Curr Med Res Opin*. 2009 Feb;25(2):401–11.

58. Ramsey SD, Liu Z, Boer R, et al. Cost-effectiveness of primary versus secondary prophylaxis with pegfilgrastim in women with early-stage breast cancer receiving chemotherapy. *Value Health*. 2009 Mar-Apr;12(2):217–25.

59. Waller EK. The role of sargramostim (rhGM-CSF) as immunotherapy. *Oncologist*. 2007 12 Suppl 2:22–6.

60. Rini BI, Fong L, Weinberg V, Kavanaugh B, Small EJ. Clinical and immunological characteristics of patients with serologic progression of prostate cancer achieving long-term disease control with granulocyte-macrophage colony-stimulating factor. *J Urol*. 2006 Jun;175(6):2087–91.

61. Kurbacher CM, Kurbacher JA, Cramer EM, et al. Continuous low-dose GM-CSF as salvage therapy in refractory

recurrent breast or female genital tract carcinoma. *Oncology (Williston Park).* 2005 Apr;19(4 Suppl 2):23–6.

62. Heaney ML, Toy EL, Vekeman F, et al. Comparison of hospitalization risk and associated costs among patients receiving sargramostim, filgrastim, and pegfilgrastim for chemotherapy-induced neutropenia. *Cancer.* 2009 Oct 15;115(20):4839–48.

63. Available at: http://www.kaiserhealthnews.org/stories/2014/june/17/insurers-push-against-cancer-treatment-cost.aspx. Accessed June 28, 2014.

64. Albright JW, Albright JF. Impaired natural killer cell function as a consequence of aging. *Exp Gerontol.* 1998 Jan-Mar;33(1–2):13–25.

65. Ogata K, Yokose N, Tamura H, et al. Natural killer cells in the late decades of human life. *Clin Immunol Immunopathol.* 1997 Sep;84(3):269–75.

66. Kmiec Z, Myśliwska J, Rachón D, Kotlarz G, Sworczak K, Myśliwski A. Natural killer activity and thyroid hormone levels in young and elderly persons. *Gerontology.* 2001 Sep-Oct;47(5):282–8.

67. Vitale M, Zamai L, Neri LM, et al. The impairment of natural killer function in the healthy aged is due to a postbinding deficient mechanism. *Cell Immunol.* 1992 Nov;145(1):1–10.

68. Di Lorenzo G, Balistreri CR, Candore G, et al. Granulocyte and natural killer activity in the elderly. *Mech Ageing Dev.* 1999 Apr 1;108(1):25–38.

69. McNerlan SE, Rea IM, Alexander HD, Morris TC. Changes in natural killer cells, the CD57CD8 subset, and related cytokines in healthy aging. *J Clin Immunol.* 1998 Jan;18(1):31–8.

70. Dussault I, Miller SC. Decline in natural killer cell-mediated immunosurveillance in aging mice-a consequence of reduced cell production and tumor binding capacity. *Mech Ageing Dev.* 1994 Aug;75(2):115–29.

71. Camous X, Pera A, Solana R, Larbi A. NK cells in healthy aging and age-associated diseases. *BioMed Research International*. 2012;2012:195956.

72. Lutz CT, Quinn LS. Sarcopenia, obesity, and natural killer cell immune senescence in aging: altered cytokine levels as a common mechanism. *Aging* (Albany NY). 2012; 4(8):535–46.

73. Wu J, Lanier LL. Natural killer cells and cancer. *Adv Cancer Res*. 2003 90:127–56.

74. Lodoen MB, Lanier LL. Natural killer cells as an initial defense against pathogens. *Curr Opin Immunol*. 2006 Aug;18(4):391–8.

75. Grégoire C, Chasson L, Luci C, et al. The trafficking of natural killer cells. *Immunol Rev*. 2007 Dec;220:169–82.

76. Vivier E, Tomasello E, Baratin M, Walzer T, Ugolini S. Functions of natural killer cells. *Nat Immunol*. 2008 May;9(5):503–10.

77. Mccoy JL, Rucker R, Petros JA. Cell-mediated immunity to tumor-associated antigens is a better predictor of survival in early stage breast cancer than stage, grade or lymph node status. *Breast Cancer Res Treat*. 2000 Apr;60(3):227–34.

78. Koda K, Saito N, Takiguchi N, Oda K, Nunomura M, Nakajima N. Preoperative natural killer cell activity: correlation with distant metastases in curatively research colorectal carcinomas. *Int Surg*. 1997 Apr-Jun;82(2):190–3.

79. Da Costa ML, Redmond P, Bouchier-Hayes DJ. The effect of laparotomy and laparoscopy on the establishment of spontaneous tumor metastases. *Surgery*. 1998 Sep;124(3):516–25.

80. Shakhar G, Ben-Eliyahu S. Potential prophylactic measures against postoperative immunosuppression: could they reduce recurrence rates in oncological patients? *Ann Surg Oncol*. 2003 Oct;10(8):972–92.

81. McCulloch PG, MacIntyre A. Effects of surgery on the generation of lymphokine-activated killer cells in patients with breast cancer. *Br J Surg*. 1993 Aug;80(8):1005–7.

82. Rosenne E, Shakhar G, Melamed R, Schwartz Y, Erdreich-Epstein A, Ben-Eliyahu S. Inducing a mode of NK-resistance to suppression by stress and surgery: a potential approach based on low dose of poly I-C to reduce postoperative cancer metastasis. *Brain Behav Immun*. 2007 May;21(4):395–408.

83. Fehniger TA, Bluman EM, Porter MM, et al. Potential mechanisms of human natural killer cell expansion in vivo during low-dose IL-2 therapy. *J Clin Invest*. 2000 Jul;106(1):117–24.

84. Caligiuri MA, Zmuidzinas A, Manley TJ, Levine H, Smith KA, Ritz J. Functional consequences of interleukin 2 receptor expression on resting human lymphocytes. Identification of a novel natural killer cell subset with high affinity receptors. *J Exp Med*. 1990 May 1;171(5):1509–26.

85. Orange JS, Roy-Ghanta S, Mace EM, et al. IL-2 induces a WAVE2-dependent pathway for actin reorganization that enables WASp-independent human NK cell function. *J Clin Invest*. 2011 Apr;121(4):1535–48.

86. Rowe JM, Andersen JW, Mazza JJ, et al. A randomized placebo-controlled phase III study of granulocyte-macrophage colony-stimulating factor in adult patients (> 55 to 70 years of age) with acute myelogenous leukemia: a study of the Eastern Cooperative Oncology Group (E1490). *Blood*. 1995 Jul 15;86(2):457–62.

87. Buchsel PC, DeMeyer ES. Dendritic cells: emerging roles in tumor immunotherapy. *Clin J Oncol Nurs*. 2006 Oct;10(5):629–40.

88. Spitler LE. Adjuvant therapy of melanoma. *Oncology* (Williston Park). 2002 Jan;16(1 Suppl 1):40–8.

89. Available at: http://www.manhattan-institute.org/html/ib_15.htm#.U7BFr2dOXDc. Accessed July 2, 2014.

90. Available at: http://www.forbes.com/sites/dougbandow/2012/06/11/end-the-fda-drug-monopoly-let-patients-choose-their-medicines/3/. Accessed July 2, 2014.

91. Peppercorn J, Burstein H, Miller FG, Winer E, Joffe S. Self-reported practices and attitudes of US oncologists regarding off-protocol therapy. *J Clin Oncol.* 2008 Dec 20;26(36):5994–6000.

92. Available at: http://www.cancer.org/treatment/treatments andsideeffects/treatmenttypes/chemotherapy/off-label-drug-use. Accessed June 23, 2014.

93. Availableat:http://www.nytimes.com/2012/10/15/opinion/a-hospital-says-no-to-an-11000-a-month-cancer-drug. html?_r=1&. Accessed July 9, 2014.

94. Available at: http://www.ajmc.com/publications/evidence-based-oncology/2012/2012-2-vol18-n5/breast-cancer-will-treatment-costs-outpace-effectiveness. Accessed July 9, 2014.

95. Available at: http://www.biomedcentral.com/content/pdf/1472-6963-11-305.pdf. Accessed July 9, 2014.

96. Available at: http://www.beckershospitalreview.com/finance/wellpoint-to-pay-monthly-bonuses-to-oncologists-who-comply-with-clinical-pathways.htm. Accessed June 24, 2014.

97. Available at: http://www.fiercepharma.com/story/cancer-drugs-beware-docs-get-monthly-paybacks-sticking-pre-ferred-meds/2014-05-28. Accessed June 24, 2014.

98. Chattopadhyay M, Kodela R, Kashfi K. P09 Therapeutic potential of NOSH-aspirin, a dual nitric oxide-and hydro-gen sulfide-donating hybrid in colon cancer. *Nitric Oxide.* 2013 Sep 1;31 Suppl 2:S37–8.

99. Fraser DM, Sullivan FM, Thompson AM, McCowan C. Aspi-rin use and survival after the diagnosis of breast cancer: a population-based cohort study. *Br J Cancer.* 2014 Jun 19.

100. Yue W, Yang CS, DiPaola RS, Tan XL. Repurposing of met-formin and aspirin by targeting AMPK-mTOR and inflam-mation for pancreatic cancer prevention and treatment. *Cancer Prev Res (Phila).* 2014 Apr;7(4):388–97.

101. Ucbek A, Ozünal ZG, Uzun O, Gepdıremen A. Effect of metformin on the human T98G glioblastoma multiforme cell line. *Exp Ther Med.* 2014 May;7(5):1285–90.

102. Zhang ZJ, Bi Y, Li S, et al. Reduced risk of lung cancer with metformin therapy in diabetic patients: a systematic review and meta-analysis. *Am J Epidemiol.* 2014 Jul 1;180(1):11–4.

103. Wang Z, Lai ST, Xie L, et al. Metformin is associated with reduced risk of pancreatic cancer in patients with type 2 diabetes mellitus: A systematic review and meta-analysis. *Diabetes Res Clin Pract.* 2014 Apr 18.

104. Fasih A, Elbaz HA, Hüttemann M, Konski AA, Zielske SP. Radiosensitization of Pancreatic Cancer Cells by Metformin through the AMPK Pathway. *Radiat Res.* 2014 Jul;182(1)50–9.

105. Queiroz EA, Puukila S, Eichler R, et al. Metformin Induces Apoptosis and Cell Cycle Arrest Mediated by Oxidative Stress, AMPK and FOXO3a in MCF-7 Breast Cancer Cells. *PLoS One.* 2014 May 23;9(5):e98207.

106. Takahashi A, Kimura F, Yamanaka A, et al. Metformin impairs growth of endometrial cancer cells via cell cycle arrest and concomitant autophagy and apoptosis. *Cancer Cell Int.* 2014 Jun 16;14:53.

107. Joshua AM, Zannella VE, Downes MR, et al. A pilot 'window of opportunity' neoadjuvant study of metformin in localised prostate cancer. *Prostate Cancer Prostatic Dis.* 2014 May 27.

108. Preston MA, Riis AH, Ehrenstein V, et al. Metformin Use and Prostate Cancer Risk. *Eur Urol.* 2014 May 21. pii: S0302-2838(14)00408-4.

109. Zhang T, Zhang L, Zhang T, et al. Metformin Sensitizes Prostate Cancer Cells to Radiation Through EGFR/p-DNA-PKCS In Vitro and In Vivo. *Radiat Res.* 2014 Jun;181(6):641–9.

110. Miyoshi H, Kato K, Iwama H, et al. Effect of the anti-diabetic drug metformin in hepatocellular carcinoma in vitro and in vivo. *Int J Oncol.* 2014 Jul;45(1):322–32.

111. Cho SW, Yi KH, Han SK, et al. Therapeutic potential of metformin in papillary thyroid cancer in vitro and in vivo. *Mol Cell Endocrinol*. 2014 Jun 3;393(1–2):24–29.

112. Yen YC, Lin C, Lin SW, Lin YS, Weng SF. Effect of metformin on the incidence of head and neck cancer in diabetes. *Head Neck*. 2014 May 7.

113. Sun XJ, Zhang P, Li HH, Jiang ZW, Jiang CC, Liu H. Cisplatin combined with metformin inhibits migration and invasion of human nasopharyngeal carcinoma cells by regulating E-cadherin and MMP-9. *Asian Pac J Cancer Prev*. 2014 15(9):4019–23.

114. Cerezo M, Tomic T, Ballotti R, Rocchi S. Is it time to test biguanide metformin in the treatment of melanoma? *Pigment Cell Melanoma Res*. 2014 May 24.

115. Nenu I, Popescu T, Aldea MD, et al. Metformin associated with photodynamic therapy-A novel oncological direction. *J Photochem Photobiol B*. 2014 May 21;138C:80–91.

116. Kantarjian H, Giles F, List A, et al. The incidence and impact of thrombocytopenia in myelodysplastic syndromes. *Cancer*. 2007 May 1;109(9):1705–14.

117. Quintás-Cardama A, Kantarjian H, Ravandi F, et al. Bleeding diathesis in patients with chronic myelogenous leukemia receiving dasatinib therapy. *Cancer*. 2009 Jun 1;115(11):2482–90.

118. Rickles FR, Falanga A, Montesinos P, Sanz MA, Brenner B, Barbui T. Bleeding and thrombosis in acute leukemia: what does the future of therapy look like? *Thromb Res*. 2007;120 Suppl 2:S99–106.

119. Avvisati G, Tirindelli MC, Annibali O. Thrombocytopenia and hemorrhagic risk in cancer patients. *Crit Rev Oncol Hematol*. 2003 Oct 15;48(Suppl):S13–6.

120. Kris MG, Johnson BE, Berry LD, et al. Using multiplexed assays of oncogenic drivers in lung cancers to select targeted drugs. *JAMA*. 2014 May 21;311(19):1998–2006.

121. Available at: http://www.mdanderson.org/newsroom/news-releases/2012/key-discovered-to-how-chemotherapy-drug-causes-heart-failure.html. Accessed July 12, 2014.

122. Available at: http://www.ncbi.nlm.nih.gov/pmc/articles/PMC2848530/. Accessed July 12, 2014.

123. Swain SM, Whaley FS, Ewer MS. Congestive heart failure in patients treated with doxorubicin: a retrospective analysis of three trials. *Cancer*. 2003 Jun 1;97(11):2869–79.

124. Delozier T, Vernhes JC. Comparative study of adriamycin, epirubicin and mitoxantrone in cancer of the breast. Review of the literature. *Bull Cancer*. 1991 Nov;78(11):1013–25.

125. Wiseman LR, Spencer CM. Mitoxantrone. A review of its pharmacology and clinical efficacy in the management of hormone-resistant advanced prostate cancer. *Drugs Aging*. 1997 Jun;10(6):473–85.

126. Henderson IC, Allegra JC, Woodcock T, et al. Randomized clinical trial comparing mitoxantrone with doxorubicin in previously treated patients with metastatic breast cancer. *J Clin Oncol*. 1989 May;7(5):560–71.

127. Available at: http://www.cancer.org/cancer/lungcancer-smallcell/detailedguide/small-cell-lung-cancer-survival-rates. Accessed July 3, 2014.

128. Available at: http://www.cancer.org/cancer/colonandrectumcancer/detailedguide/colorectal-cancer-survival-rates. Accessed July 3, 2014.

129. Available at: http://www.cancer.org/cancer/breastcancer/detailedguide/breast-cancer-survival-by-stage. Accessed July 3, 2014.

130. Available at: http://webreprints.djreprints.com/3405331420659.html. Accessed July 3, 2014.

131. Soderberg-Naucler C, Rahbar A, Stragliotto G. Survival in patients with glioblastoma receiving valganciclovir. *NEJM*. Sep 5 2013;369(10):985–6.

132. Dziurzynski K, Chang SM, Heimberger AB, et al. Consensus on the role of human cytomegalovirus in glioblastoma. *Neuro Oncol.* 2012 Mar 14(3):246–55.

133. Barami K. Oncomodulatory mechanisms of human cytomegalovirus in gliomas. *J Clin Neurosci.* 2010 July 17(7):819–23.

134. Soroceanu L, Cobbs CS. Is HCMV a tumor promoter? *Virus Res.* 2011 May 157(2):193–203.

135. Available at: http://www.cdc.gov/cmv/overview.html. Accessed June 26, 2014.

136. Available at: http://www.webmd.com/cancer/brain-cancer/news/20130904/antiviral-drug-may-extend-brain-cancer-survival-researchers-say. Accessed June 26, 2014.

137. Available at: http://www.lef.org/magazine/mag2014/apr2014_Unsustainable-Cancer-Drug-Prices_01.htm. Accessed June 30, 2014.

138. Available at: http://ir.wellpoint.com/phoenix.zhtml?c=130104&p=irol-newsArticle&ID=1934999&highlight. Accessed June 30, 2014.

139. Available at: http://www.imshealth.com/portal/site/imshealth/menuitem.c76283e8bf81e98f53c753c71ad8c22a/?vgnextoid=19b381d71adc5410VgnVCM10000076192ca2RCRD&vgnextfmt=default. Accessed June 30, 2014.

Intolerable Delays!

T HE FIRST SURGICAL ATTEMPT to cure pancreatic cancer was demonstrated in Germany in 1909.[1]

In 1935, a doctor named Allen Whipple devised a more effective way to remove the pancreas and adjacent body parts.[2] Dr. Whipple's technique involves the removal of the head of the pancreas, along with portions of the stomach, small intestine, gall bladder, and common bile duct. The surgical impact on the body is severe. There is a higher death rate from this procedure than many other hospital operations.[3] Sometimes the rearranged internal organs do not hold together and infection spreads inside the patient. This leads to follow-up surgery where the remainder of the pancreas and the spleen are removed to correct problems caused by the first operation.[4]

Some patients do not heal well and leak pancreatic juice from where body parts are sewn together. This happens so frequently that the surgeon leaves in drainage catheters for fluids to exit so they don't accumulate inside the patient.[4,5] Another complication is paralysis of the stomach that can take over a month to heal. During this time, a feeding tube is surgically placed into the small intestine to provide nourishment.[6] Some patients develop type I diabetes because the insulin-producing areas of their pancreas are removed, requiring life-long insulin injections.[7] Despite these horrific surgical side effects, most patients who survive the painful hospital ordeal die from metastatic pancreatic cancer. Few are cured.

The name of this surgery is the "Whipple Procedure." While it's been refined since Dr. Whipple's work in 1935, pancreatic cancer is still killing the vast majority of its victims—79 years later![8] The snail's pace of progress against malignancies like pancreatic cancer should provoke societal outrage against the establishment. Yet like lambs standing in line awaiting slaughter, the public tolerates mediocre medicine that is inflicting horrific suffering and massive numbers of needless deaths. We view these bureaucratic lags as intolerable delays that will be ridiculed by future medical historians. This chapter describes a drug long ago approved by the FDA that can improve outcomes in pancreatic and other cancer cases. This treatment, however, is not being incorporated into conventional practice.

Steve Jobs was criticized for delaying a Whipple Procedure for nine months after being diagnosed with pancreatic cancer.[9] The initial approaches Jobs tried (acupuncture, vegan diet, herbs, spiritualists) had no chance of eradicating his primary pancreatic tumor. It's hard to blame the then 49-year-old co-founder of Apple, however, for not wanting his body cut up via a Whipple Procedure. Steve Jobs eventually died at age 56 after undergoing multiple aggressive treatments, including a liver transplant.[10–12]

How many technologies developed in the early 1900s do consumers still use today? Even the stethoscope (invented in 1819) remains state-of-the-art in today's archaic world of medical practice. If one is diagnosed with pancreatic cancer at a relatively early stage, the Whipple Procedure is still the best treatment option. Overlooked are myriad adjuvant therapies that can markedly improve long-term survival and reduce the horrific complications inherent to the Whipple surgical procedure. The cancer treatment I describe next is not new. It has long been recommended to Life Extension® members.

INTERLEUKIN-2 VERSUS PLACEBO IN PANCREATIC CANCER TREATMENT

The subcutaneous administering of 9 million international units a day of the drug interleukin-2 to pancreatic cancer patients three days <u>before</u> surgery induced the following benefits compared to placebo patients administered saline:

	Interleukin-2 Group	Control
Two-Year Survival	33%	10%
Three-Year Survival	22%	0%
Postoperative Complications	33%	80%

This study should have made headline news. Instead it was buried in a 2006 edition of the journal *Hepato-Gastroenterology*.[46] Life Extension® has been recommending moderate dose interleukin-2 as an adjuvant cancer treatment since the late 1990s.

Skeptics point to studies in advanced melanoma and renal cell carcinoma patients where interleukin-2 provides only modest survival improvements. These narrow-focused cynics neglect evidence that interleukin-2 is most effective when administered before immune-suppressing surgery, radiation, and chemotherapy begins.[33–37,47,48]

INTERLEUKIN-2 IMPROVES SURVIVAL 3-FOLD!

Interleukin-2 (IL-2) enhances overall immune function, most notably by enhancing natural killer cell activity.[13-15] Natural killer cells are among the body's most important immune defenses against malignant and viral-infected cells.[16-20] (Cells infected with certain viruses are more prone to convert to malignant cells.)[21] IL-2 was long ago approved to treat kidney cancer[22-26] and metastatic melanoma.[27-29] Its efficacy was likely limited by the advanced disease stage patients are at by the time IL-2 is administered.[30] There is toxicity associated with high-dose IL-2.[31,32]

Intriguing research suggests that administering moderate-dose IL-2 to patients before surgery and chemotherapy may improve survival and other outcomes.[33-37] It does this by boosting immune function prior to it being impaired by conventional treatments. Surgery results in significant immune impairment, something we warned against long before the mainstream considered it a factor in the poor survival rates seen in many types of cancer.[38-43] Immune suppression that occurs during chemotherapy is a well-established treatment complication.[44,45]

In a study conducted on pancreatic cancer patients, half the group was administered moderate dose IL-2 for three consecutive days prior to a Whipple Procedure. Two years after the operation, 33% of patients pre-administered IL-2 were alive compared to only 10% of control surgical patients. Three-year survival was 22% in the IL-2 group compared to 0% of the controls.[46]

Surgical complications occurred in 80% of the control surgical patients compared with only 33% in the IL-2 pretreatment group. While the control group spent 19.5 days confined to the hospital after their Whipple Procedure, the IL-2 group escaped the hospital in 12 days.[46]

Life Extension® has been recommending moderate-dose IL-2 since the 1990s, yet the mainstream oncologists behave as if these drugs are limited to advanced cancers for which they originally gained FDA approval. The reality is that IL-2 and other immune-boosting drugs may have far greater efficacy when administered early in the disease process against of a wide range of solid tumors and some types of leukemia.

WHY CANCER PATIENTS NEED TO BOOST NATURAL KILLER CELL ACTIVITY

Natural killer cells are the part of the immune system that is capable of recognizing and killing virus-infected and malignant cells, while sparing normal cells.[49,50]

The importance of killing virus-infected cells is that cells infected with human papilloma virus (HPV) and other viruses have greater propensity to mutate into cancer cells. Chronic infection with some of these viruses also exhausts vital immune functions.[51]

In mice deficient in natural killer cells, tumors grow more aggressively and are more metastatic.[52–54]

Natural killer cells play an important role in the control of tumor growth.[55]

Infusion of immune enhancers like interleukin-2 boosts natural killer cell activity, which can lead to the death of tumor cells.[56]

Leukemia patients have benefited using natural killer cells obtained from hematopoietic stem cell donors, which is an exciting area of cancer research.[57–59]

Non-drug ways of boosting natural killer cell activity include garlic,[60–64] melatonin,[65–67] Reishi extract,[68–71] and other supplements used by Life Extension® clients. When treating cancer, however, interleukin-2 should be considered to provide an exponential improvement in natural killer cell activity prior to initiation of conventional treatments.

CONTRAST MEDIOCRE CANCER TREATMENT TO HIV

Cancer is not relegated to modern times. It has killed human beings forever, but has become prominent as people live longer and cancer incidence markedly increases. Pancreatic cancer, for instance, increases sharply in individuals over age 50, and most patients are 60 to 80 years old when diagnosed.[72]

HIV rose to prominence in the early 1980s, though the virus existed in the human population before then. The problem was that no one paid attention until thousands started dying.

Within 15 years of HIV infection becoming pandemic, effective anti-viral "cocktails" were discovered that turned AIDS from a death sentence into a manageable chronic disease.[73–75]

In 1981, AIDS was a disease of unknown origin.[76] It is controllable today because of rapid scientific innovation. Pancreatic cancer, on the other hand, still kills virtually all its victims with the best hope for long-term survival being the Whipple Procedure first refined in 1935.[8]

So why were AIDS treatments discovered so quickly while effective cancer therapies languish?

The difference was the aggressive way that experimental multi-modal therapies were implemented in HIV/AIDS patients compared to the suffocating bureaucracy that stymies cancer research.

In the early days of AIDS treatment, any therapy that might work was tried immediately on dying patients and the results evaluated and documented. These treatments were often administered by those infected with HIV who faced pending death if a cure were not discovered quickly. The FDA was cast by the wayside as AIDS activists made certain that potentially effective treatments were not obstructed by bureaucratic red tape.[77]

We at Life Extension® are proud of the part we played in saving the lives of AIDS patients by defying FDA attempts to shut us down. An editorial published late last year in the *New England Journal of Medicine* revealed how HIV revolutionized the way global health is pursued, and how it resulted in accelerated delivery of innovative life-saving treatments.[78]

NEW ENGLAND JOURNAL OF MEDICINE PRAISES WORK OF EARLY AIDS ACTIVISTS

Allan Brandt, PhD, is a professor of medical history at Harvard Medical School. Dr. Brandt's perspective, titled "How AIDS Invented Global Health," was published in the June 6, 2013 edition of the *New England Journal of Medicine*.[79] Here are some quotes from his perspective:

- "AIDS has reshaped conventional wisdoms in public health, research practice, cultural attitudes, and social behaviors."

- "The rapid development of effective antiretroviral treatments, in turn, could not have occurred without new forms of disease advocacy and activism."

- "But AIDS activists explicitly crossed a vast chasm of expertise. They went to FDA meetings and events steeped in often arcane science of HIV, prepared to offer concrete proposals to speed research, reformulate trials, and accelerate regulatory processes."

- "This approach went well beyond the traditional bioethical formulations of autonomy and consent. As many clinicians and scientists acknowledged, AIDS activists, including many people with AIDS, served as collaborators and colleagues rather than constituents and subjects, changing the trajectory of research and treatment."

Omitted from Dr. Brandt's complimentary statements were the harassment, persecution, and incarceration of AIDS activists by government agencies that sought to suppress burgeoning development of AIDS therapies.[80,81]

WE WERE JAILED!

The FDA did not like our aggressive stance when it came to accelerating medical research, particularly as it related to helping AIDS victims. The FDA did everything in its power to shut Life Extension® down and imprison us for life.[82] According to the FDA, we were ripping off dying AIDS patients by recommending unproven therapies.

The *Journal of the American Medical Association* (November 27, 2013) featured an article describing a 54% reduction in the risk of progressing from HIV to full-blown AIDS using selenium and multi-vitamins.[83] Life Extension® first recommended these nutrients in the October 1985 edition of the *Life Extension Magazine* (called at that time *Anti-Aging News*). While the study published in the *Journal of the American Medical Association* was conducted in a region of Africa where malnutrition is rampant, and the study had other flaws (like a 25% dropout rate in both groups), the delay in HIV-induced immune suppression in patients taking these nutrients was remarkable. A number of previous studies support the benefits of certain nutrients in delaying HIV progression[79,84–86] Even *FDA Consumer Magazine* eventually acknowledged the value of AIDS patients using nutrient supplements.

We also recommended a drug called isoprinosine to AIDS patients in the October 1985 issue of *Anti-Aging News*. This contributed to our being arrested by the FDA because isoprinosine was not an approved drug. In the June 21, 1990 edition of the *New England Journal of Medicine*, a study found that HIV-infected humans who took isoprinosine were eight times less likely to progress to AIDS compared to placebo.[87] This was not enough, however, to keep us from being indicted in 1991. What helped save us was the continuing publication of research findings corroborating that isoprinosine and certain nutrients significantly delayed disease progression in HIV-infected patients, thus negating the FDA's argument that we were "ripping off AIDS patients" by recommending "unproven" therapies.

The FDA was on the wrong side when it sought to destroy us in the 1980s–1990s. Regrettably, millions of Americans continue to perish from needless bureaucratic red tape from virtually all diseases except AIDS. The reason AIDS is the exception is that AIDS activists made it clear to the FDA that there would be no bureaucratic delays in delivering experimental therapies to HIV-infected patients. The FDA capitulated and this enabled rapid medical innovation to occur in a free-market environment.

Cancer patients, on the other hand, sit by like timid sheep, as the FDA decides which experimental therapy they are "allowed" to try and how far their disease must progress before the experimental therapy is made available on a so-called "compassionate-use" basis. FDA's granting of "compassionate-use" sometimes occurs weeks after the patient dies, or is so close to death that it has no chance of working.

In conclusion, our data suggest the relevance of NK (natural killer) cells as primary effectors not only against high-risk leukemias, but also solid tumors. [44]*

NOT FAST ENOUGH!

In 2010, the Life Extension Foundation® pledged a substantial amount of money to a prestigious cancer research institute to evaluate many of the components contained in our published "Pancreatic Cancer Treatment Protocol." The institution eagerly pushed this project forward, generating reams of paperwork in order to obtain Institutional Review Board approval. By 2014, the total number of pancreatic patients enrolled in this study is zero. Bureaucratic delays like this are beyond rational understanding. These are human lives we are talking about!

When we devised unique treatments for AIDS in the 1980s, they were provided to dying AIDS patients almost overnight. Not all of them worked, but the ones that did built on a foundation that has resulted in HIV patients living for decades, as opposed to pancreatic cancer patients who often die in a matter of months. Contrast the rapid development of AIDS therapies to most pancreatic cancer patients who die even after enduring the Whipple Procedure that was first described in 1935. It is clear that methods employed by AIDS activists are far superior to today's regulatory quagmire that stymies cancer research.

---

* Quote from study published in the April 2013 edition of the journal *Oncoimmunology*.

CITIZENS SHOULD REVOLT

Cancer will likely kill over 570,000 Americans this year.[88] Already-approved treatments could be saving lives, such as administering moderate dose interleukin-2 early in the disease process. Yet even these simple treatment enhancements are ignored by the oncology mainstream that prefers to practice assembly line medicine. These kinds of delays would have never been tolerated by AIDS activists, who experimented with any potentially effective drug on large numbers of dying patients to quickly discover what worked and what didn't.

The *New England Journal of Medicine* credits the work of AIDS pioneers as revolutionizing the way medical research is conducted today. We at Life Extension® disagree with this Pollyanna assessment, as cancer therapies we uncovered decades ago remain bogged down in FDA red tape. Many are not being pursued at all despite a continuous stream of favorable data flowing out of research facilities. The slogan below was chanted by AIDS activists who surrounded FDA headquarters in 1988 and shut down the agency for one day:[89,90]

"Act Up, Speak Out . . . Silence = Death!"

PROTEST NOW RATHER THAN WAIT FOR FUNERALS

I do not know why every cancer patient and their family does not march on Washington to demand the same exemption from bureaucratic suffocation that enabled HIV to become a manageable disease in a relatively brief window of time. Perhaps cancer patients should write their family and friends and state something to the effect:

> In lieu of attending my funeral, would you mind marching on the Capitol in Washington, DC, and insist that cancer patients have unfettered access to any therapy that might work?

References

1. Specht G, Stinshoff K. Walther Kausch (1867–1928) and his significance in pancreatic surgery. *Zentralbl Chir.* 2001 Jun;126(6):479–81.

2. Available at: http://www.grandroundsjournal.com/articles/gr07l0001/gr07l0001.pdf. Accessed March 6 , 2014.

3. Birkmeyer JD, Siewers AE, Finlayson EV, et al. Hospital volume and surgical mortality in the United States. *N Engl J Med.* 2002 Apr 11;346(15):1128–37.

4. Ho CK , Kleeff J,Friess H, Büchler MW. Complications of pancreatic surgery. *HPB (Oxford).* 2005;7(2):99–108.

5. Shrikhande SV, D'Souza MA. Pancreatic fistula after pancreatectomy: evolving definitions, preventive strategies and modern management. *World J Gastroenterol.* 2008 Oct 14;14(38):5789–96.

6. Wente MN, Bassi C, Dervenis C, et al. Delayed gastric emptying (DGE) after pancreatic surgery: a suggested definition by the International Study Group of Pancreatic Surgery (ISGPS). *Surgery.* 2007 Nov;142(5):761–8.

7. Ferrara MJ, Lohse C, Kudva YC, et al. Immediate post-resection diabetes mellitus after pancreaticoduodenectomy: incidence and risk factors. *HPB (Oxford).* 2013 Mar;15(3):170–4.

8. Available at: http://www.webmd.com/cancer/pancreatic-cancer/whipple-procedure. Accessed March 6, 2014.

9. Available at: http://money.cnn.com/2008/03/02/news/companies/elkind_jobs.fortune/index.htm?postversion=2008030510. Accessed March 6, 2014.

10. Available at: http://www.forbes.com/sites/erikkain/2011/10/05/steve-jobs-has-died-at-age-56/. Accessed March 6, 2014.

11. Available at: http://abcnews.go.com/Health/CancerPrevention AndTreatment/steve-jobs-pancreatic-cancer-timeline/story?id=14681812. Accessed March 6, 2014

12. Available at: http://usatoday30.usatoday.com/news/ health/medical/health/medical/cancer/story/2011-08-24/ Apple-CEO-Steve-Jobs-resigns-after-battling-pancreatic-cancer/50127460/1. Accessed March 6, 2014.

13. Weigent DA, Stanton GJ, Johnson HM. Interleukin 2 enhances natural killer cell activity through induction of gamma interferon. *Infect Immun.* 1983 Sep;41(3):992–7.

14. Kehrl JH, Dukovich M, Whalen G, Katz P, Fauci AS, Greene WC. Novel interleukin 2 (IL-2) receptor appears to mediate IL-2-induced activation of natural killer cells. *J Clin Invest.* 1988 Jan;81(1):200–5.

15. Yao HC, Liu SQ, Yu K, Zhou M, Wang LX. Interleukin-2 enhances the cytotoxic activity of circulating natural killer cells in patients with chronic heart failure. *Heart Vessels.* 2009 Jul;24(4):283–6.

16. Yokoyama WM, Altfeld M, Hsu KC. Natural killer cells: tolerance to self and innate immunity to viral infection and malignancy. *Biol Blood Marrow Transplant.* 2010 Jan;16(1 Suppl):S97–S105.

17. Hwang I, Scott JM, Kakarla T, et al. Activation mechanisms of natural killer cells during influenza virus infection. *PLoS One.* 2012 7(12):e51858.

18. Brandstadter JD, Yang Y. Natural killer cell responses to viral infection. *J Innate Immun.* 2011;3(3):274–9.

19. Chisholm SE, Reyburn HT. Recognition of vaccinia virus-infected cells by human natural killer cells depends on natural cytotoxicity receptors. *J Virol.* 2006 Mar;80(5):2225–33.

20. Viel S, Charrier E, Marçais A, et al. Monitoring NK cell activity in patients with hematological malignancies. *Oncoimmunology.* 2013 Sep 1;2(9):e26011.

21. zur Hausen H. Immortalization of human cells and their malignant conversion by high risk human papillomavirus genotypes. *Semin Cancer Biol.* 1999 Dec;9(6):405–11.

22. Rosenberg SA, Lotze MT, Muul LM, et al. Observations on the systemic administration of autologous lymphokine-activated killer cells and recombinant interleukin-2 to patients with metastatic cancer. *N Engl J Med.* 1985 Dec 5;313(23):1485–92.

23. Salup RR, Wiltrout RH. Adjuvant immunotherapy of established murine renal cancer by interleukin 2-stimulated cytotoxic lymphocytes. *Cancer Res.* 1986 Jul;46(7):3358–63.

24. Marumo K, Ueno M, Muraki J, Baba S, Tazaki H. Augmentation of cell-mediated cytotoxicity against renal carcinoma cells by recombinant interleukin 2. *Urology.* 1987 Oct;30(4):327–32.

25. Wang J, Walle A, Gordon B, et al. Adoptive immunotherapy for stage IV renal cell carcinoma: a novel protocol utilizing periodate and interleukin-2-activated autologous leukocytes and continuous infusions of low-dose interleukin-2. *Am J Med.* 1987 Dec;83(6):1016–23.

26. Fisher RI, Coltman CA Jr, Doroshow JH, et al. Metastatic renal cancer treated with interleukin-2 and lymphokine-activated killer cells. A phase II clinical trial. *Ann Intern Med.* 1988 Apr;108(4):518–23.

27. Chu MB, Fesler MJ, Armbrecht ES, et al. High-dose interleukin-2 (HD IL-2) therapy should be considered for the treatment of patients with melanoma brain metastases. *Chemother Res Pract.* 2013 2013:726925.

28. Atkins MB, Kunkel L, Sznol M, Rosenberg SA. High-dose recombinant interleukin-2 therapy in patients with metastatic melanoma: long-term survival update. *Cancer J Sci Am.* 2000 Feb;6 Suppl 1:S11–4.

29. Keilholz U, Conradt C, Legha SS, et al. Results of interleukin-2-based treatment in advanced melanoma: a case record-based analysis of 631 patients. *J Clin Oncol.* 1998 Sep;16(9):2921–9.

30. Petrella T, Quirt I, Verma S, et al. Single-agent interleukin-2 in the treatment of metastatic melanoma. *Curr Oncol.* 2007 Feb;14(1):21–6.

31. Acquavella N, Kluger H, Rhee J, et al. Toxicity and activity of a twice daily high-dose bolus interleukin 2 regimen in patients with metastatic melanoma and metastatic renal cell cancer. *J Immunother*. 2008 Jul-Aug;31(6):569–76.

32. Schwartz RN, Stover L, Dutcher J. Managing toxicities of high-dose interleukin-2. *Oncology*. 2002 Nov;16(11 Suppl 13):11–20.

33. Brivio F, Lissoni P, Rovelli F, et al. Effects of IL-2 preoperative immunotherapy on surgery-induced changes in angiogenic regulation and its prevention of VEGF increase and IL-12 decline. *Hepatogastroenterology*. 2002 Mar-Apr;49(44):385–7.

34. Böhm M, Ittenson A, Klatte T, et al. Pretreatment with interleukin-2 modulates perioperative immunodysfunction in patients with renal cell carcinoma. *Folia Biol (Praha)*. 2003 49(2):63–8.

35. Nichols PH, Ramsden CW, Ward U, Sedman PC, Primrose JN. Perioperative immunotherapy with recombinant interleukin 2 in patients undergoing surgery for colorectal cancer. *Cancer Res*. 1992 Oct 15;52(20):5765–9.

36. Lissoni P, Brivio F, Fumagalli L, Di Fede G, Brera G. Enhancement of the efficacy of chemotherapy with oxaliplatin plus 5-fluorouracil by pretreatment with IL-2 subcutaneous immunotherapy in metastatic colorectal cancer patients with lymphocytopenia prior to therapy. *In Vivo*. 2005 Nov-Dec;19(6):1077–80.

37. Ades EW, McKemie CR 3rd, Wright S, Peacocke N, Pantazis C, Lockhart WL 3rd.Chemotherapy subsequent to recombinant interleukin-2 immunotherapy: protocol for enhanced tumoricidal activity. *Nat Immun Cell Growth Regul*. 1987 6(5):260–8.

38. Da Costa ML, Redmond P, Bouchier-Hayes DJ. The effect of laparotomy and laparoscopy on the establishment of spontaneous tumor metastases. *Surgery*. 1998 Sep;124(3):516–25.

39. Shakhar G, Blumenfeld B. Glucocorticoid involvement in suppression of NK activity following surgery in rats. *J Neuroimmunol*. 2003 May;138(1–2):83–91.

40. Rosenne E, Shakhar G, Melamed R, Schwartz Y, Erdreich-Epstein A, Ben-Eliyahu S. Inducing a mode of NK-resistance to suppression by stress and surgery: a potential approach based on low dose of poly I-C to reduce postoperative cancer metastasis. *Brain Behav Immun*. 2007 May;21(4):395–408.

41. Marik PE, Flemmer M. The immune response to surgery and trauma: Implications for treatment. *J Trauma Acute Care Surg*. 2012 Oct;73(4):801–8.

42. Yokoyama Y, Sakamoto K, Arai M, Akagi M. Radiation and surgical stress induce a significant impairment in cellular immunity in patients with esophageal cancer. *Jpn J Surg*. 1989 Sep;19(5):535–43.

43. Sano T, Morita S, Tominaga R, et al. Adaptive immunity is severely impaired by open-heart surgery. *Jpn J Thorac Cardiovasc Surg*. 2002 May;50(5):201–5.

44. Rasmussen L, Arvin A. Chemotherapy-induced immunosuppression. *Environ Health Perspect*. 1982 Feb;43:21–5.

45. Zandvoort A, Lodewijk ME, Klok PA, et al. After chemotherapy, functional humoral response capacity is restored before complete restoration of lymphoid compartments. *Clin Exp Immunol*. 2003 Jan;131(1):8–16.

46. Angelini C, Bovo G, Muselli P, et al. Preoperative interleukin-2 immunotherapy in pancreatic cancer: preliminary results. *Hepatogastroenterology*. 2006 Jan-Feb;53(67):141–4.

47. Hietanen T, Kellokumpu-Lehtinen P, Pitkänen M. Action of recombinant and interleukin 2 in modulating radiation effects on viability and cytotoxicity of large granular lymphocytes. *Int J Radiat Biol*. 1995 Feb;67(2):119–26.

48. Boise LH, Minn AJ, June CH, Lindsten T, Thompson CB. Growth factors can enhance lymphocyte survival without committing the cell to undergo cell division. *Proc Natl Acad Sci U S A*. 1995 Jun 6;92(12):5491–5.

49. Oberoi P, Wels WS. Arming NK cells with enhanced anti-tumor activity: CARs and beyond. *Oncoimmunology*. 2013 Aug 1;2(8):e25220.

50. Sanchez-Correa B, Morgado S, Gayoso I, Bergua JM, Casado JG, Arcos MJ, Bengochea ML, Duran E, Solana R, Tarazona R. Human NK cells in acute myeloid leukaemia patients: analysis of NK cell-activating receptors and their ligands. *Cancer Immunol Immunother*. 2011 Aug;60(8):1195–205.

51. Brunner S, Herndler-Brandstetter D, Weinberger B, Grubeck-Loebenstein B. Persistent viral infections and immune aging. *Ageing Res Rev*. 2011 Jul;10(3):362–9.

52. Kozlowski JM, Fidler IJ, Campbell D, Xu ZL, Kaighn ME, Hart IR. Metastatic behavior of human tumor cell lines grown in the nude mouse. *Cancer Res*. 1984 Aug;44(8):3522–9.

53. Kim S, Iizuka K, Aguila HL, Weissman IL, Yokoyama WM. In vivo natural killer cell activities revealed by natural killer cell-deficient mice. *Proc Natl Acad Sci USA*. 2000 Mar 14;97(6):2731–6.

54. Smyth MJ, Swann J, Cretney E, Zerafa N, Yokoyama WM, Hayakawa Y. NKG2D function protects the host from tumor initiation. *J Exp Med*. 2005 Sep 5;202(5):583–8.

55. Vacca P, Martini S, Mingari MC, Moretta L. NK cells from malignant pleural effusions are potent antitumor effectors: A clue for adoptive immunotherapy? *Oncoimmunology*. 2013 Apr 1;2(4):e23638.

56. Bhat R, Watzl C. Serial killing of tumor cells by human natural killer cells—enhancement by therapeutic antibodies. *PLoS One*. 2007 Mar 28;2(3):e326.

57. Bradstock KF. The use of hematopoietic growth factors in the treatment of acute leukemia. *Curr Pharm Des*. 2002 8(5):343–55.

58. Ruggeri L, Mancusi A, Burchielli E, Aversa F, Martelli MF, Velardi A. Natural killer cell alloreactivity in allogeneic hematopoietic transplantation. *Curr Opin Oncol*. 2007 Mar;19(2):142–7.

59. Locatelli F, Pende D, Mingari MC, et al. Cellular and molecular basis of haploidentical hematopoietic stem cell transplantation in the successful treatment of high-risk leukemias: role of alloreactive NK cells. *Front Immunol.* 2013 Feb 1;4:15.

60. Ishikawa H, Saeki T, Otani T, et al. Aged garlic extract prevents a decline of NK cell number and activity in patients with advanced cancer. *J Nutr.* 2006 Mar;136(3 Suppl):816S-20S.

61. Nantz MP, Rowe CA, Muller CE, Creasy RA, Stanilka JM, Percival SS. Supplementation with aged garlic extract improves both NK and gd-T cell function and reduces the severity of cold and flu symptoms: a randomized, double-blind, placebo-controlled nutrition intervention. *Clin Nutr.* 2012 Jun;31(3):337–44.

62. Tang Z, Sheng Z, Liu S, Jian X, Sun K, Yan M. [The preventing function of garlic on experimental oral precancer and its effect on natural killer cells, T-lymphocytes and interleukin-2]. *Hunan Yi Ke Da Xue Xue Bao.* 1997 22(3):246–8.

63. Kyo E, Uda N, Suzuki A, et al. Immunomodulation and antitumor activities of Aged Garlic Extract. *Phytomedicine.* 1998 Aug;5(4):259–67.

64. Butt MS, Sultan MT, Butt MS, Iqbal J. Garlic: nature's protection against physiological threats. *Crit Rev Food Sci Nutr.* 2009 Jun;49(6):538–51.

65. Miller SC, Pandi-Perumal SR, Esquifino AI, Cardinali DP, Maestroni GJ. The role of melatonin in immuno-enhancement: potential application in cancer. *Int J Exp Pathol.* 2006 Apr;87(2):81–7.

66. Currier NL, Miller SC. Echinacea purpurea and melatonin augment natural-killer cells in leukemic mice and prolong life span. *J Altern Complement Med.* 2001 Jun;7(3):241–51.

67. Srinivasan V, Spence DW, Pandi-Perumal SR, Trakht I, Cardinali DP. Therapeutic actions of melatonin in cancer: possible mechanisms. *Integr Cancer Ther*. 2008 Sep;7(3):189–203.

68. Lin ZB. Cellular and molecular mechanisms of immunomodulation by Ganoderma lucidum. *J Pharmacol Sci*. 2005 Oct;99(2):144–53.

69. Gao Y, Zhou S, Jiang W, Huang M, Dai X. Effects of ganopoly (a Ganoderma lucidum polysaccharide extract) on the immune functions in advanced-stage cancer patients. *Immunol Invest*. 2003 Aug;32(3):201–15.

70. Zheng S, Jia Y, Zhao J, Wei Q, Liu Y. Ganoderma lucidum polysaccharides eradicates the blocking effect of fibrinogen on NK cytotoxicity against melanoma cells. *Oncol Lett*. 2012 Mar;3(3):613–16.

71. Zhu XL, Lin ZB. Effects of Ganoderma lucidum polysaccharides on proliferation and cytotoxicity of cytokine-induced killer cells. *Acta Pharmacol Sin*. 2005 Sep;26(9):1130–7.

72. Bast RC Jr, Kufe DW, Pollock RE, et al., editors. Holland-Frei Cancer Medicine. 5th edition. Hamilton (ON): BC Decker; 2000. Available at: http://www.ncbi.nlm.nih.gov/books/NBK20889/.

73. Arts EJ, Hazuda DJ. HIV-1 antiretroviral drug therapy. *Cold Spring Harb Perspect Med*. 2012 Apr;2(4):a007161.

74. De Clercq E. Anti-HIV drugs: 25 compounds approved within 25 years after the discovery of HIV. *Int J Antimicrob Agents*. 2009 Apr;33(4):307–20.

75. Sahay S, Reddy KS, Dhayarkar S. Optimizing adherence to antiretroviral therapy. *Indian J Med Res*. 2011 Dec;134(6):835–49.

76. Adler MW. ABC of Aids: Development of the epidemic. *BMJ*. 2001 May 19;322(7296):1226–9.

77. Available at: http://www.fda.gov/ForConsumers/ByAudience/ForPatientAdvocates/HIVandAIDSActivities/ucm258087.htm. Accessed March 6, 2014.

78. Available at: http://www.nejm.org/doi/full/10.1056/ NEJMp1305297. Accessed March 14, 2014.

79. Fawzi WW, Msamanga GI, Spiegelman D, et al. A randomized trial of multivitamin supplements and HIV disease progression and mortality. *N Engl J Med.* 2004 Jul 1;351(1):23–32.

80. [No authors listed] AIDS advocates returning to their activism roots. Protesters welcome arrests and publicity. AIDS Alert. 2004 Aug;19(8):90–3.

81. Available at: http://www.tcnj.edu/~borland/2006-aids/cassy2. htm Accessed March 14, 2014.

82. Available at:http://www.lef.org/magazine/mag2003/oct2003_ cover_victory_01.htm. Accessed March 14, 2014.

83. Baum MK, Campa A, Lai S, et al. Effect of micronutrient supplementation on disease progression in asymptomatic, antiretroviral-naive, HIV-infected adults in Botswana: a randomized clinical trial. *JAMA.* 2013 Nov 27;310(20):2154–63.

84. Fawzi WW, Msamanga GI, Kupka R, et al. Multivitamin supplementation improves hematologic status in HIV-infected women and their children in Tanzania. *Am J Clin Nutr.* 2007 May;85(5):1335–43.

85. Botros D, Somarriba G, Neri D, Miller TL. Interventions to address chronic disease and HIV: strategies to promote exercise and nutrition among HIV-infected individuals. *Curr HIV/ AIDS Rep.* 2012 Dec;9(4):351–63.

86. Mehta S, Fawzi W. Effects of vitamins, including vitamin A, on HIV/AIDS patients. *Vitam Horm.* 2007 75:355–83.

87. Pedersen C, Sandström E, Petersen CS, et al. The efficacy of inosine pranobex in preventing the acquired immunodeficiency syndrome in patients with human immunodeficiency virus infection. The Scandinavian Isoprinosine Study Group. *N Engl J Med.* 1990 Jun 1;322(25):1757–63.

88. Available at: http://www.cdc.gov/nchs/fastats/deaths.htm. Accessed March 17, 2014.

89. Available at: http://theconversation.com/how-the-dallas-buyers-club-changed-hiv-treatment-in-the-us-22664. Accessed March 17, 2014.

90. Available at: http://www.edgeboston.com/health_fitness/hiv_aids/News//154077/act-up_co-f. Accessed March 17, 2014.

DECEMBER 2011

Bureaucratic Assault on New Cancer Therapies

O NE AMERICAN DIES EVERY HOUR from melanoma.[1] Incidences of this deadly skin cancer are on the increase. Although no cure exists for advanced melanoma, virtually 100% of its victims can be saved if the malignancy is caught early.[2] The problem is that dermatologists cannot accurately diagnose a melanoma based on a visual examination alone. A biopsy is needed to definitely ascertain if a skin lesion is a melanoma. Biopsies require expenditure of money and time, along with some minor trauma. Patients and dermatologists have to make decisions as to whether a particular skin lesion warrants a biopsy.

In a clinical trial involving 23 dermatologists around the US, a hand-held non-invasive scanning device called MelaFind® was tested on suspicious lesions. Its accuracy in detecting melanoma was 98%—which equaled or bested the top doctors in avoiding unnecessary biopsies.[3] MelaFind® was submitted for FDA approval in June 2009. Despite clinical trial results documenting its unprecedented (98%)

ability to detect early stage melanoma, the FDA refused to approve it and insisted on further review.[4,5]

FDA'S LETHAL ILLOGIC

According to bureaucratic illogic, the FDA was concerned that non-dermatologists might use MelaFind® to screen for melanoma, even though the company promised to only sell it to dermatologists. Since the FDA cannot regulate doctors, the agency felt that the best way of keeping MelaFind® out of the hands of non-dermatologists was to not approve it at all.

The FDA expressed other concerns such as its misuse by dermatologists. This is rather bizarre since dermatologists are the most highly trained in our society to diagnose and treat skin diseases, yet the FDA did not want them to use this new device that was 98% accurate in diagnosing melanoma.[6,7]

THE REAL WORLD OF MEDICAL PRACTICE

FDA bureaucrats live in a cave when it comes to the intricacies and expenses involved in the real-world medical setting. Hurried people too often ignore suspicious skin lesions until it's too late. Patients often go to their primary care doctor when it comes to suspicious skin lesions. More enlightened individuals visit a dermatologist. Either way, medical efficiency comes into play when deciding whether a suspicious lesion should be biopsied or merely kept an eye on. A dermatologist charges for each biopsy, and there is a separate expense for the pathology lab. Return visits are often needed. All this adds up to medical costs that MelaFind® could otherwise render far more efficient.

MelaFind® is not 100% accurate. That means it may miss a few (2%) suspicious lesions that a dermatologist would then have to decide warranted a biopsy nonetheless. The FDA is using this as another reason not to approve it. Using this logic, MRI and ultrasound testing would never have been approved because these are not 100% reliable diagnostic tools either.

If ever approved, MelaFind® will provide doctors with an efficient method to detect early stage melanoma. According to some dermatologists, it has the potential to "save many lives."[8] There were 68,130 new cases of melanoma in 2010 and 8,700 deaths.[9] These numbers show that melanoma can be easily cured—if caught in the early stages before it infiltrates and metastasizes. We at Life Extension® envision a day when devices like MelaFind® will be used in large screening campaigns where early stage melanomas can be easily detected and removed. None of this will happen as long as the FDA is allowed to erect bureaucratic barriers that suppress this kind of medical innovation.

FDA APPROVES EXPENSIVE MELANOMA DRUG

Cynical individuals might question the timing of the FDA's denial of MelaFind®, a device that could spare thousands of agonizing deaths from metastatic melanoma. Just a few weeks after saying no to MelaFind®, the FDA approved a new drug by pharmaceutical giant Bristol-Meyers Squibb to treat advanced melanoma trademarked Yervoy™.[10] In a study involving 676 patients with advanced melanoma, those receiving Yervoy™ survived for 10 months compared to 6.4 months for those who did not receive it. Fourteen patients died from side effects caused by Yervoy™.[11] The FDA hailed this as a breakthrough and granted approval for widely spread melanoma.

Shares of Bristol-Meyers Squibb surged as analysts predicted a $1.7 billion blockbuster.[12] The reason so much money will be made is that it will cost each patient an astounding

$120,000 for the four-course treatment.[4] For what used to be the price of a nice home, one with terminal melanoma can buy an extra 108 days of life. The average cost per day of added life will be over $1,000—further exacerbating today's healthcare cost crisis!

The generic name for Yervoy™ is ipilimumab. If you ever wonder why you cannot pronounce the names of new compounds (like ipilimumab), it is because pharmaceutical companies intentionally create names that no one can readily comprehend. Pharmaceutical companies do this to make it harder for future generic drug makers to enter the market with lower-cost versions, since virtually no one can pronounce the generic name.

The reason that Yervoy™ (ipilimumab) is expected to sell so well is that current FDA-approved therapies have not been shown to substantially extend survival, but the FDA allowed them to be used for decades anyway. We are not against the FDA's approval of Yervoy™ as it may prove to work better when treating less advanced melanoma. What bothers us are the bureaucratic barriers. They are so cumbersome that few new therapies ever get approved. This enables companies to charge extortionist prices for the few that receive the FDA's coveted anointment.

FDA FAILS TO APPROVE EFFECTIVE LYMPHOMA DRUG

Each year about 65,000 Americans are diagnosed with non-Hodgkin lymphoma.[13] It is estimated to have killed over 20,000 in the US in 2010. Jackie Kennedy Onassis died from non-Hodgkin lymphoma at the age of 64.[15] Non-Hodgkin lymphoma is one of the few cancers where establishment medicine can brag about treatment breakthroughs. Over the past 50 years, survival rates have more than doubled.[16] Often overlooked are long-term side effects like cumulative heart muscle damage that precludes long-term use of certain conventional treatments.[17] Lymphoma patients who fail treatment with FDA-approved chemotherapy have a life expectancy measured in weeks or months.

A next-generation compound called pixantrone is designed to be less toxic and more effective than current anthracycline chemo drugs. It has successfully gone through phase I and phase II human clinical trials. In 2004, a randomized phase III trial mandated by the FDA was initiated. Pixantrone was administered to non-Hodgkin lymphoma patients who had already failed conventional therapy. The control group received whatever their oncologist thought would work best for them. In these extremely difficult-to-treat lymphoma patients, 20% of those receiving pixantrone showed a complete response, compared to only 6% receiving conventional care.[18] A follow-up analysis of the data showed 24% of patients attaining complete response status as opposed to 7% in the standard group.[19] These are unprecedented findings!

A complete response is not a cure, but it can buy a patient precious time in remission and the opportunity to identify potential curative therapies. Despite almost four years of phase III clinical studies showing that pixantrone works three times better than what's available today, the FDA declined to approve it. In an FDA briefing as to why pixantrone was not approved, the FDA stated, "The study was not stopped at a planned interim analysis and early study stopping invalidated the applicant's Special Protocol Assessment."[20] The "Special Protocol Assessment" is an agreement between the FDA and a drug maker regarding how a clinical study should be done.[21] It originally envisioned enrolling 320 patients over a 36-month time period. For various reasons, it took 45 months to recruit 140 patients.[22] This is not unusual as some 60% of phase III studies do not meet patient recruitment objectives, but nonetheless generate statistically significant data that are used to approve a new drug.

PIXATRONE NOT OWNED BY BIG PHARMA

Unlike Bristol-Meyers Squibb, which had the wherewithal to fund a huge clinical study and whose stock soared in response to the FDA's approval of Yervoy™,[23] the maker of pixantrone's auditors handed management a notice that the company (Cell Therapeutics) may not be able to continue as a going concern in response to the FDA's refusal to approve their drug.[24,25] Cell Therapeutics' initial challenge in enrolling enough study subjects was convincing oncologists and hematologists that pixantrone might work. Patient incentive to participate was minimized because the FDA mandated that only 50% of the study subjects would receive the promising drug (pixantrone).

Despite these limitations, Cell Therapeutics believes it generated statistically significant data and has taken the unusual step of appealing the FDA's denial of pixantrone. The reason appeals are seldom filed is fear of FDA retaliation on future drug applications. In the case of Cell Therapeutics, which is not part of Big Pharma, it may have little to risk in asking for a common-sense review of the impressive data it generated in terminally ill lymphoma patients. The inability of Cell Therapeutics to adhere to the FDA's impossible-to-achieve dictates is an example of a federal agency that went out of its way to railroad a promising cancer therapy.

HOW LIFE EXTENSION® IS HELPING TO ACCELERATE MELANOMA TREATMENT

Scientists supported by the Life Extension Foundation® long ago discovered a novel method of treating advanced melanoma (stages 3 and 4). In an FDA-approved clinical trial, a topical cream (called imiquimod) is applied to the exposed tumor twice a day for a total of six weeks. At weeks two and four, the doctors expose the area to an infrared laser. The topical imiquimod cream binds with receptors on cancer cells and stimulates them to activate proteins that "broadcast" the presence of the tumor cells to the immune system. In essence, the patient's own tumor cells become a unique anti-tumor vaccine. The laser portion of the treatment is designed to hyperactivate the imiquimod with the objective of inducing a systemic immune response against metastatic melanoma cells.

This same protocol is being done in the Bahamas for melanoma, and a modified version is being studied to treat breast cancer. In order for this treatment to be administered, a tumor lesion must be present near the surface of your skin, such as a breast lump, a chest wall breast lesion, or a superficial melanoma tumor. To inquire about clinical programs being offered in the Bahamas, call the International Strategic Cancer Alliance (ISCA) at 610-628-3419 or visit www.iscanceralliance.com.

THE REAL ISSUE . . .

The way this country tolerates FDA behavior, it is as if only large pharmaceutical companies are capable of discovering effective new drugs. Those without deep pockets are often shut out of today's Byzantine approval process, where it can cost over $100 million to have a new compound "approved" for sale. Most troubling is what this is doing to medical innovation across the entire spectrum. We at Life Extension® know of pioneering physicians who have discovered and are utilizing novel therapeutic protocols to treat the diseases of aging. Yet these inventions have virtually no chance of making it out of these private practices because of FDA overregulation.

To see how much more efficient an unregulated environment functions, look no further than the breakthroughs that have been made in the treatment of AIDS. This disease appeared in America around 1980. It took several years just to identify the HIV virus as the cause. In the first half of the 1980s, virtually everyone who contracted AIDS died within 1–2 years. The difference was that AIDS activists were acutely aware that FDA-mandated randomized clinical trials were the roadblock to the discovery of effective therapies. Unlike cancer support groups who too often capitulate to FDA suppression, AIDS activists rebelled and forced the FDA to back down from restricting any therapy that might be effective.

Removed from the artificial constraints of controlled trials designed by uncaring and incompetent bureaucrats, frontline doctors and researchers were able to collect data from actual medical practice on AIDS patients and had the flexibility of trying whatever therapy might work. Life Extension® partnered with these groups early on and witnessed the miraculous results that occurred when doctors could prescribe therapies without regard to FDA dictates. When Life Extension® attempted to introduce this same strategy to dying cancer patients, the FDA stood in the way and said absolutely not!

LOW CoQ10 LEVELS ASSOCIATED WITH 790% INCREASED RISK OF MELANOMA METASTASIS

In a study published in the *Journal of the American Academy of Dermatology*, plasma coenzyme Q10 levels were measured in 117 consecutive melanoma patients upon enrollment. 125 matched volunteers without any clinically suspected pigmented lesions were utilized as the control group. Researchers found that CoQ10 levels were significantly lower in melanoma patients compared to control subjects. Further, it was noted that for melanoma patients with CoQ10 blood levels of less than 0.6 mg per liter, the risk of developing metastatic disease increased by 790%, compared to those melanoma patients with blood levels of 0.6 mg per liter or higher. In addition, melanoma patients with higher blood levels had a metastasis-free interval that was almost double compared to patients with lower levels.[29]

Of the 82 patients with low CoQ10 levels, 17 died during the study, compared to none of the 35 patients with higher CoQ10. CoQ10 levels did not vary by sex.[29] Levels of CoQ10 correlated well with tumor thickness, which is currently the best indicator of melanoma progression. Specifically, lower CoQ10 levels correlated with increased tumor thickness and poorer prognosis.[29] The study notes that abnormally low plasma levels of CoQ10 previously have been known in patients with cancer of the breast, lung, and pancreas. This study may be the first to indicate that lower blood levels of CoQ10 can have an extremely adverse effect. The lead author of the study concluded that analysis of their findings suggested baseline CoQ10 levels are a powerful and independent prognostic factor that can be used to estimate risk for melanoma progression.

Statin drugs are known to lower CoQ10 levels. Will we find that melanoma progression is another side effect of statins? If so, this side effect can be readily overcome with CoQ10 supplements.

LOOK AT THE DIFFERENCE BETWEEN AIDS AND CANCER

Those afflicted with AIDS today are prescribed an armamentarium of medications and take huge quantities of dietary supplements to keep their infections under control. What used to be a near-certain death sentence has turned into a manageable chronic disease for most people. That happened more than a decade ago! Contrast this with cancer, where a melanoma drug that gives patients an extra 108 days of life (that costs $120, 000)[10] is hailed as a breakthrough in 2011. Americans have been dying of melanoma for hundreds of years. The FDA's approval of expensive and mediocre drugs like Yervoy™ and suppression of common-sense approaches (like MelaFind® and pixantrone) are stark examples of the FDA's bureaucratic assault on novel cancer therapies.

At the June 2011 conference of the American Society of Clinical Oncology (ASCO), the results from several human studies were announced about new compounds that prolong the lives of advanced melanoma patients.[26] Despite an unusual amount of enthusiasm shown by oncology researchers, it may take years before the FDA will allow combinations of these compounds to be used in desperately ill melanoma patients . . . who are dying at the rate of one each hour. One of the new targeted melanoma drugs featured at the June ASCO meeting is called vemurafenib and is being developed by Roche Holding AG and Daiichi Sankyo's Plexxikon unit. It inhibits a mutated form of a gene called BRAF found in more than half of patients with advanced melanoma. It has virtually no benefit on patients with a normal version of the gene. Results from a 675-patient trial showed that those taking vemurafenib were 63% less likely to die over a six-month period compared to those taking chemotherapy called dacarbazine.[28] The median time before the disease progressed for patients on vemurafenib was 5.3 months compared with 1.6 months on dacarbazine chemotherapy.

Based on this trial, we believe that melanoma patients with a mutated BRAF gene should have been allowed immediate access to vemurafenib if they were willing to sign a disclaimer acknowledging that it is not yet FDA-approved. Instead, thousands of melanoma patients are dying prematurely in the FDA's waiting room.

MY GRANDMOTHER'S FUNERAL

At age 13, I stood over the casket of my grandmother, who had died a horrific death from melanoma. She was only 54 and suffered terribly as metastatic lesions invaded every part of her body. Her death was preventable, as she ignored a melanoma lesion on her leg for many years. At that funeral in 1968, no one would have predicted that more Americans than ever would be dying of melanoma in 2011—43 years later! Like others back then, our family believed that medicine would advance and find a cure for cancer, just like antibiotics wiped out most bacterial infections.

While major technological advances are routine in virtually all disciplines, clinical medicine is the exception. It has devolved into a bureaucratic monstrosity that suffocates innovation while rewarding the politically well-connected. How much longer will Americans tolerate a system that is a proven failure?

As My Article Was Being Finalized . . . FDA Partially Capitulates on MelaFind®

In response to intense legal and political pressure put on the FDA, a limited conditional approval has just been granted for the MelaFind® skin cancer detection device.[30] This pending approval comes after a seven-year battle between the company that makes MelaFind® and the FDA. After FDA rejected MelaFind® last year, the company filed a citizen's petition with FDA Commissioner Margaret Hamburg seeking to overturn the denial.

The House of Representatives held a hearing in the summer of 2011 where the FDA's top device regulator acknowledged the agency mishandled the MelaFind® application. The error occurred when the FDA denied approval of MelaFind® before it held a meeting of its own scientific advisors—talk about bureaucratic mix-up! This does not mean that MelaFind® will definitely become available, but the FDA is at least moving off its refusal to approve it at all. MelaFind® did win approval in early September in 27 European nations.

In order for MelaFind® to be approved in the US, the FDA needs to agree on the device's final labeling, a user guide, details of a training program for doctors, and the design of a post-approval clinical trial. The CEO of the company that makes MelaFind® was uncertain about when the FDA would approve MelaFind® and was careful to downplay if and when the company can begin selling the device. He acknowledged that discussions with the FDA were still going "back and forth" and therefore not complete. Before MelaFind® can be sold in the US, the FDA wants additional "beta tests" with doctors to be conducted to make technical and usability improvements to the device. The FDA insists that MelaFind's label be longer and more complicated than the company ever envisioned. Until these issues are resolved, MelaFind® will not be allowed on the American market.

There are examples of other products in the past that received this kind of conditional FDA approval but never made it to the market, though it seems the political heat has forced the FDA in a direction regarding MelaFind® that it previously refused to consider. If you ever wonder why medical advances take so long and then cost so much, the expense and delay in pushing MelaFind® through the FDA's cumbersome bureaucracy provides a stark example.

References

1. Available at: http://www.melanomafoundation.org/facts/statistics.htm. Accessed May 18, 2011.

2. Available at: http://www.projectmelanoma.com/a-national-challenge.php. Accessed May 18, 2011.

3. Monheit G, Cognetta AB, Ferris L, et al. The performance of MelaFind: a prospective multicenter study. Arch Dermatol. 2011 Feb;147(2):188–94.

4. Available at: http://www.marketwire.com/press-release/MELA-Sciences-Announces-FDA-Panel-Review-MelaFind-PMA-Application-on-August-26-2010-NASDAQ-MELA-1266362.htm. Accessed May 18, 2011.

5. Available at: http://www.thestreet.com/story/10944267/3/biotech-calendar-fda-drug-approvals-in-2011.html. Accessed May 18, 2011.

6. Available at: http://www.medpagetoday.com/Dermatology/SkinCancer/23448. Accessed May 19, 2011.

7. Available at: http://www.modernmedicine.com/modern medicine/Modern+Medicine+Now/MelaFind-device-raises-concerns-among-some-dermato/ArticleStandard/Article/detail/706390. Accessed May 19, 2011.

8. Available at: http://online.wsj.com/article/SB10001424052 748704559904576230562290013904.html. Accessed May 20, 2011.

9. Available at: http://seer.cancer.gov/statfacts/html/melan.html. Accessed May 20, 2011.

10. Available at: http://www.bloomberg.com/news/2011-03-25/bristol-myers-squibb-wins-u-s-fda-approval-for-new-melanoma-medicine.html. Accessed May 20, 2011.

11. Hodi FS, O'Day SJ, McDermott DF, et al. Improved survival with ipilimumab in patients with metastatic melanoma. N Engl J Med. 2010 Aug 19;363(8):711–23.

12. Available at: http://www.mmm-online.com/fda-approves-bms-skin-cancer-biologic-yervoy/article/199258/. Accessed May 21, 2011.

13. Available at: http://www.non-hodgkins-lymphoma-cancer.org/news/non-hodgkins-news0026.htm. Accessed May 20, 2011.

14. Available at: http://seer.cancer.gov/statfacts/html/nhl.html. Accessed May 23, 2011.

15. Available at: http://www.nytimes.com/learning/general/onthisday/bday/0728.html Accessed May 23, 2011.

16. Available at: http://www.lls.org/diseaseinformation/getinformationsupport/factsstatistics/nonhodgkinlymphoma/. Accessed May 23, 2011.

17. Available at: http://www.drugs.com/health-guide/non-hodgkin-lymphoma.html. Accessed May 24, 2011.

18. Available at: http://www.drugs.com/clinical_trials/cell-therapeutics-pixantrone-phase-iii-extend-pivotal-trial-successful-achieving-primary-endpoint-6168.html. Accessed May 24, 2011.

19. Available at: http://www.fda.gov/downloads/advisorycommittees/committeesmeetingmaterials/drugs/oncologicdrugsadvisorycommittee/ucm199560.pdf. Accessed May 25, 2011.

20. Available at: http://online.wsj.com/article/SB10001424052748703766704576009512990553104.html. Accessed May 26, 2011.

21. Available at: http://www.fda.gov/downloads/AdvisoryCommittees/CommitteesMeetingMaterials/Drugs/OncologicDrugsAdvisoryCommittee/UCM204335.pdf. Accessed May 26, 2011.

22. Available at: http://www.pharmalot.com/2010/02/the-fda-and-special-protocal-assessments/. Accessed May 26, 2011.

23. Available at: http://www.bloomberg.com/news/2011-03-25/
bristol-myers-squibb-wins-u-s-fda-approval-for-new-
melanoma-medicine.html. Accessed May 30, 2011.

24. Available at: http://seekingalpha.com/article/198401-fda-
s-early-verdict-on-cell-therapeutics-pixuvri-comes-as-no-
surprise. Accessed May 30, 2011.

25. Available at: http://www.ipdatadepot.com/archives/
ipp070402.pdf. (pg. 13/45). Accessed May 30, 2011.

26. Available at: http://online.wsj.com/article/SB1000142405
27023044323045763678025809935000.html?mod=WSJ_
hp_MIDDLENexttoWhatsNewsTop. Accessed May 31, 2011.

27. Available at: http://www.bloomberg.com/news/2011-05-
25/roche-leads-deadly-skin-cancer-turnaround-as-dozen-
drugs-coming.html. Accessed May 31, 2011.

28. Chapman PB, Hauschild A, Robert C, et al. Improved survival with vemurafenib in melanoma with BRAF V600E
mutation. N Engl J Med. 2011 Jun 10 30;364(26);2507–16.

29. Rusciani L, Proietti I, Rusciani A, et al. Low plasma coenzyme
Q10 levels as an independent prognostic factor for melanoma
progression. J Am Acad Dermatol. Feb 2006;54(2):234–41.

30. Burton TJ. New tool in skin-cancer fight. FDA reversal clears
path for a device that helps doctors diagnose melanoma.
Wall Street Journal. September 26, 2011.

Cancer Establishment Hides Radiation Side Effects

I N A SHOCKING EXPOSÉ of the cancer establishment, Dr. Ralph Moss in his frequently updated book *The Cancer Industry* revealed the sordid history of radiation therapy. The first victims were researchers and physicians who succumbed to radiation's lethal effects without even suspecting it posed a danger to them. The next set of medical victims was patients who received severe burns from radiation overdoses that left them painfully mutilated or dead from acute radiation poisoning. As radiation doses were refined, the cancer establishment proclaimed a major treatment breakthrough. Yet the statistics were manipulated to cover up what was really happening to irradiated patients. For instance, patients with progression-free survival of 5 years (or less) are often listed as successes even if the same cancer later returns.[1,2]

Most disturbing are statistical methods that ignore lethal side effects such as radiation necrosis in the brain that kills the majority of its victims, but are not always officially tabulated as cancer deaths.[3,4] This enables statisticians to say the radiation "cured" the patient of cancer, while omitting the fact that the therapy itself killed the patient. Radiation therapy is an important part of treating certain head and neck tumors and is often used after surgery,[5] but lethal radiation necrosis to the brain is one potential side effect.[6] Radiation therapy is routinely used to treat primary brain tumors. The cure rate for the most common brain tumors is disturbingly low,[7] but even in those fortunate enough to have their brain tumors destroyed by the radiation, a large percentage succumb shortly thereafter to radiation necrosis of the brain.[8]

The more prevalent and omitted cover-up relates to the long-term impact of radiation therapy. For example, another danger of radiation therapy to the head is increased risk of stroke.[9] A study of head and neck cancer patients who received radiation therapy found that stroke rates were five times greater than expected.[10] This elevated stroke risk was found many years after administration of radiation. The average time between radiation treatment and stroke was 10.9 years, but the increased risk of stroke persisted for 15 years after radiation therapy. For cancer patients treated with radiation therapy that later die from a stroke, the official cause of death is stroke, even though the radiation therapy often caused the stroke. This is an example of how cancer cure statistics are misleading. The government contends that radiation therapy is curing cancer patients, yet long-term radiation side effects cause many deaths that are not attributed to cancer.

The government claims that more cancer victims are living beyond five years, but ignores the fact that the toxic therapies used to eradicate cancer can themselves cause premature death.[11]

High-dose radiation to the chest cavity increases heart disease risk . . . and this side effect may not occur for 20 years or later.[12] Some of the side effects from radiation therapy to the breast include a breakdown of the skin or such severe pain in the breast that surgery is needed for treatment.[13] Radiation therapy given to the axillary lymph nodes can increase the risk of patients developing arm swelling ("lymphedema") following axillary (armpit) dissection.[14–17] Radiation to this area can cause numbness, tingling, or even pain and loss of strength in the hand and arm years after treatment.[14,16] Some patients develop "radiation pneumonitis," a lung reaction that causes a cough, shortness of breath, and fevers three to nine months after completing treatment.[16] These side effects may go away within a relatively short time or persist over an extended period.

The primary concern with radiation therapy is that it may initiate secondary cancers years or decades after the primary cancer was "cured." This does not mean that all cancer patients should refuse radiation therapy, as it often adds years or decades to their lives, and is in many cases curative. But as Ralph Moss, PhD, graphically described in his *Cancer Industry* books, oncology researchers are motivated to achieve complete responses that they can later claim to be cancer "cures." Overlooked from the statistics are horrific long-term side effects that leave patients permanently mutilated, in constant pain with loss of bodily functions, and under chronic medical care to deal with the damage inflicted by the "cancer cure." Patients suffering side effects from conventional treatments are often never the same again, yet the cancer establishment uses these cases to create statistical models to pretend their toxic therapies are a panacea.

In Suzanne Somers' case, she has long regretted her sub-mission to radiation therapy after her lumpectomy. While she made the right choice in saying "no" to chemotherapy, she has suffered for ten years from the destructive effects caused by the intense amount of radiation delivered to her breast and surrounding tissues.

HOW RADIATION CAUSES LONG-TERM DAMAGE TO BREAST TISSUES

Radiation therapy has long been used to treat breast can-cer. For patients who choose breast-conserving surgery, have multiple positive lymph nodes, or have a local recur-rence, radiation therapy will likely be part of the treat-ment plan. Radiation acts directly on the cell nucleus. Cancer cells grow rapidly compared to normal cells, so by radiating the cancerous area, cancer cells are damaged and many of them destroyed. Unfortunately, radiation also has a negative effect on normal cells. By mutating genes in the nucleus of healthy cells, these normal cells are more likely to later develop into cancer.

This damage to genes in the cells' nucleus also causes the expression of pro-inflammatory factors that result in a constant bombardment (inflammatory fires) by one's immune cytokines against the irradiated cells. As the cells initially damaged by radiation are destroyed, the "inflammatory fires" spread to nearby healthy cells and create a chain reaction whereby more healthy cells come under chronic cytokine-inflammatory attack. Radiation damages the blood supply to normal skin at a microscopic level. This results in a significantly greater risk of compli-cations following surgery. These risks include infection, delayed healing, wound breakdown, and fat necrosis, as well as implant-related problems.[18] Radiation therapy can be the source of serious problems when it comes to breast reconstruction.

THIS EXPLAINS WHY SUZANNE SOMERS STATED:

> There should be a book written on the realities of radiation and all the things that are never mentioned beforehand. With radiation, the breast gradually gets flatter and flatter until it looks as though there has been a complete mastectomy . . . when the swelling subsided it was considerably smaller than I had at first realized, and then it (Suzanne's breast) began to degrade, gradually losing more and more volume until it became non-existent.

IMPORTANT SUMMARY

This chapter is not meant to dissuade cancer patients from utilizing radiation therapy, as when properly used against specific tumors it can produce significantly higher cure rates that offset the risk of side effects. For instance, if you are diagnosed with Hodgkin lymphoma in the chest cavity, radiation has a high probability of curing you. Even though your risk of heart disease increases because of the radiation, it can buy you decades of additional life and you can take assertive steps to reduce your odds of suffering a heart attack knowing that you are at increased risk.[12,19–21] Same for stroke risk in those who receive radiation to the head. Aggressive stroke prevention may enable you to avoid the five-fold increase in stroke risk caused by the radiation.[10,22,23]

For women with breast cancer, there are established criteria for determining if radiation therapy is likely to provide a benefit that offsets the side effect risks. A careful analysis of one's individual breast cancer that includes primary tumor molecular profiling, tumor size, lymph node involvement, presence of circulating tumor cells, whole-body PET scans and CT scans, and many other diagnostics are critical to determining if radiation therapy is an appropriate choice.

Life Extension® published an extensive Cancer Radiation Protocol long ago that provides validated methods of improving the ability of radiation to eradicate cancer cells, while sparing healthy cells from radiation's many potential side effects. One can access the most recent version of the Cancer Radiation Protocol by logging on to www.lef.org/radiation_therapy. If you have any questions on the scientific content of this chapter, please call a Life Extension® Health Advisor at 1-866-864-3027.

References

1. Available at: http://www.cancer.org/Treatment/Survivorship DuringandAfterTreatment/UnderstandingRecurrence/

2. WhenYourCancerComesBack/when-cancer-comes-back-common-questions-about-recurrence. Accessed September 28, 2011.

3. Available at: http://www.cancer.net/patient/All+About+Cancer/Newly+Diagnosed/Understanding+Survival+Statistics. Accessed September 28, 2011.

4. Wang X, Hu C, Eisbruch A. Organ-sparing radiation therapy for head and neck cancer. Nat Rev Clin Oncol. 2011 Jul 26.

5. Welch HG, Black WC. Are deaths within 1 month of cancer-directed surgery attributed to cancer? J Natl Cancer Inst. 2002 Jul 17;94(14):1066–70.

6. Hunter SE, Scher RL. Clinical implications of radionecrosis to the head and neck surgeon. Curr Opin Otolaryngol Head Neck Surg. 2003 Apr;11(2):103–6.

7. Eisbruch A, Dawson L. Re-irradiation of head and neck tumors. Benefits and toxicities. Hematol Oncol Clin North Am. 1999 Aug;13(4):825–36.

8. Available at: http://emedicine.medscape.com/article/1156220-overview. Accessed October 5, 2011.

9. Available at: http://emedicine.medscape.com/article/1157533-overview. Accessed October 5, 2011.

10. Abayomi OK. Neck irradiation, carotid injury and its consequences. Oral Oncol. 2004 Oct;40(9):872–8.

11. Dorresteijn LD, Kappelle AC, Boogerd W, et al. Increased risk of ischemic stroke after radiotherapy on the neck in patients younger than 60 years. J Clin Oncol. 2002 Jan 1;20(1):282–8.

12. Lassen UN, Osterlind K, Hirsch FR, Bergman B, Dombernowsky P, Hansen HH. Early death during chemotherapy in patients with small-cell lung cancer: derivation of a prognostic index for toxic death and progression. Br J Cancer. 1999 Feb;79(3–4):515–9.

13. Boivin JF, Hutchison GB, Lubin JH, Mauch P. Coronary artery disease mortality in patients treated for Hodgkin's disease. Cancer. 1992 Mar 1;69(5):1241–7.

14. Meric F, Buchholz TA, Mirza NQ, et al. Long-term complications associated with breast-conservation surgery and radiotherapy. Ann Surg Oncol. 2002 Jul;9(6):543–9.

15. Kissin MW, Della Rovere GQ, Easton D, Westbury G. Risk of lymphodema following treatment of breast cancer. Br J surg.1986;73:580–84.

16. Stahlberg CI, Jorgensen T. Arm morbidity after axillary dissection for breast cancer. Ugeskr Laeger. 2001 Jun 11;163(24):3356–9.

17. Available at: http://www.radiologyinfo.org/en/info.cfm?pg=breastcancer#part_seven. Accessed September 29, 2011.

18. Warmuth MA, Bowen G, Prosnitz LR, et al. Complications of axillary lymph node dissection for carcinoma of the breast: a report based on a patient survey. Cancer. 1998 Oct 1;83(7):1362–8.

19. Available at: http://www.breastreconstruction.org/Recon structionOverview/RadiationandReconstruction.html. Accessed September 30, 2011.

20. Mert M, Arat-Ozkan A, Ozkara A, Aydemir NA, Babalik E. Radiation-induced coronary artery disease. Z Kardiol. 2003 Aug;92(8):682–5.

21. De Backer G, Ambrosioni E, Borch-Johnsen K, et al. European guidelines on cardiovascular disease prevention in clinical practice. Third Joint Task Force of European and other societies on cardiovascular disease prevention in clinical practice (constituted by representatives of eight societies and by invited experts). Arch Mal Coeur Vaiss. 2004 Oct;97(10):1019–30.

22. Davis W. A new paradigm for stroke prevention. *Life Extension Magazine®*. 2005 Apr;11(4):30–8.

23. Yu JG, Zhou RR, Cai GJ. From hypertension to stroke: mechanisms and potential prevention strategies. CNS Neurosci Ther. 2011 Oct;17(5):577–84.

24. Ozner M. The great American heart hoax. *Life Extension Magazine®*. 2009 May;15(5):42–8.

Taking Action

Prescription Drug Prices Surge

I N THE **FEBRUARY 2000** ISSUE of *Life Extension Magazine®* I wrote an editorial about high drug prices titled "Are We to Become Serfs of the Drug Monopoly?"

My article ignited a firestorm of activity in Congress aimed squarely at the FDA.

Back then, many members of Congress were upset that the FDA prohibited Americans from importing lower cost medications from other countries. To underscore this consumer rip-off, I compiled a chart showing how much more Americans were paying for pharmaceuticals compared to Europeans. The same chart also showed that the cost of the active drug ingredient was virtually nothing compared to what consumers had to pay.

This chart was enlarged by a congressman and shown on the floor of the House of Representatives. The purpose was to educate other lawmakers about the magnitude of the price gouging American farce.[1] The eventual result was passage of a bill by Congress and signed into law by President Bill Clinton. The bill allowed Americans to import prescription medications from countries that sold them at a fraction of the price Americans were paying.

The bill had one fatal loophole. If the FDA determined that it lacked the resources to ensure the safety of imported drugs, then the Secretary of Health and Human Services could nullify the bill with one stroke of a pen. And that's exactly what Donna Shalala did on December 27, 2000 during the final (lame-duck) month of Bill Clinton's term. This cruel act of sabotage by an unelected bureaucrat set the stage for the staggering increases in drug prices that now make headline news.

The burden of high medical costs has reached a point that is *unsustainable* by the American economy. This problem will not abate until the public regains some control over Congress, which is currently controlled by pharmaceutical lobbyists. As you'll read in this chapter, the FDA wants to further benefit pharmaceutical interests by suffocating innovation in the dietary supplement industry.

THE CURRENT CRISIS

No one has fought longer or harder against high drug prices than Life Extension®.[2] We've exposed how off-patent generic drugs whose active ingredient costs only pennies are sold to desperate consumers for hundreds of dollars. We have shown that this price gouging is caused by *over-regulation* of the prescription drug marketplace.

What's sparked recent media outrage is that the health-care burden now falls squarely on the shoulders of middle-class America.[3] That represents the majority of citizens who are facing severe economic hardships via high medical insurance premiums, high deductibles, and restricted access to the best doctors.

MAGNITUDE OF PROBLEM

There was a time not so long ago where most employers paid 100% of their employee's health insurance premiums. This included the spouse and children of each employee. If a serious medical issue arose, the company-paid insurance covered virtually 100% of the expenses. There was no such thing as first having to pay a large deductible, or being told of denial of coverage for a physician-prescribed therapy, or even denial of payment to the physician you chose.

Employees today pay a growing percentage of their own medical insurance premiums and usually 100% for their spouse and children. (Recall this was a free employee benefit just a few decades ago.) In today's upside down world of so-called health "insurance," the middle class is often limited to using physicians only in their insurance company's narrow "network." These physicians relinquish decision-making regarding diagnostics and prescribing to what the insurance company permits, which is often sub-standard care based on Life Extension's comprehensive treatment protocols.

Before the insurance company covers anything, a deductible has to be paid out-of-pocket that can easily run $4,000–$6,000. This deductible must be paid every year for treating the same medical condition. (Deductibles vary considerably depending on the plan chosen.)

So what used to be a benefit for most working Americans is now a farce. The typical working person does not run up $4,000–$6,000 in medical expenses. So they may wind up paying 100% of the healthcare costs they do incur out-of-pocket—even though they are paying higher health insurance premiums!

High co-pays (ranging from 10%-40%) even *after* the annual deductible is met mean that the middle class cannot afford to fall ill, especially as skyrocketing premiums for sub-standard insurance depletes their savings. (Low-income individuals are eligible for government subsidies to offset many of these costs, which mean they are borne instead by taxpayers.)

ALARMING NEW REPORTS

A report published in 2016 by the Brookings Institute revealed the nightmare facing middle-income Americans. The findings showed that middle-income household spending on healthcare has risen 25% from 2007 to 2014.[4] The only reason the middle-class has survived this sharp price increase is that the costs of other necessities have plummeted during that same time period.

A Kaiser Family Foundation report confirmed this bleak picture. Deductibles for individual workers have risen 67% since 2010, which is roughly 7 times more than earnings growth over the same period.[5] A separate Kaiser analysis of tens of millions of insurance claims found that patient "cost-sharing" has skyrocketed since 2004. This has been driven by a 256% surge in deductibles that consumers now have to bear.[6] Recall in the not-so-distant-past when deductibles were only a few hundred dollars.

With many generic drugs now costing thousands of dollars, and some new medications costing $100,000 each year, it is clear that only the wealthy or very poor have affordable access to healthcare in America.

Very low-income individuals have Medicaid coverage, which usually pays 100% of medical costs, even for expensive drugs that exceed $100,000 annually.

Like those with today's substandard insurance, however, Medicaid recipients are refused treatment by some of the better physicians. They at least don't have to pay out their life savings in premiums and deductibles only to be told by their insurance carrier that the therapy they need to live is "not medically necessary" or "not approved by the FDA for their specific indication."

These two excuses are routinely used by insurance carriers to deny seriously ill people access to drugs that published studies indicate are efficacious. This healthcare cost crisis is projected to worsen as employers increasingly shift more healthcare costs to workers.

WHY GENERIC DRUG PRICES ARE SKYROCKETING

Back in 2003, it cost less than $1 million to file a generic drug application with the FDA. That price was way too high as most generics can easily copy the branded drug and deliver the same bioequivalence.[11]

Today's cost of gaining FDA approval of a generic is $5 million and sometimes much higher. As a result of these oppressive approval costs, many generic drugs face no competition. This results in consumers paying almost as much as the patented version.

Excessive regulatory burdens have resulted in new generics being delayed for years while the costs of making them have been needlessly driven up by regulatory burdens. None of this excludes the probability of collusion among certain generic makers, as many cease producing a generic even after paying the costs of FDA approval. This sometimes happens when one company pays another to cease production, at which time the remaining generic propels upwards in price.

CHART PUBLISHED BY LIFE EXTENSION® IN 1999 EXPOSING SCANDALOUS HIGH DRUG PRICES*

OUTRAGEOUSLY HIGH DRUG PRICES

When we established the FDA Museum in 1994, one of the areas of malfeasance we exposed was the inflated prices Americans pay for their medicines compared to citizens of other countries. In March 1999, The Life Extension Foundation® conducted a survey of popular European and US drug prices to see what the actual difference was. We compared these drugs brand name to brand name. We are reprinting the following chart to show just how badly Americans are being defrauded by the FDA-protected drug cartel:

Drug	Potency	US Price	European Price
Premarin®	28 0 .6 mg	$14.98	$4.25
Synthroid®	50 100 mg	$13.84	$2.95
Coumadin®	25 10 mg	$30.25	$2.85
Prozac®	14 20 mg	$36.12	$18.50
Prilosec®	20 28 mg	$109.00	$39.25
Norvasc®	30 5 mg	$44.00	$23.00
Claritin®	20 10 mg	$44.00	$8.75
Augmentin®	12 500 mg	$49.50	$8.75
Zocor®	28 20 mg	$96.99	$45.00
Paxil®	28 30 mg	$63.69	$43.00
Zestril®	28 0.6 mg	$53.49	$15.00
Prempro®	50 850 mg	$23.49	$4.75
Glucophage®	60 5 mg	$54.49	$4.50
Cipro®	20 500 mg	$87.99	$62.75

* (This problem has exponentially worsened since then)

Drug	Potency	US Price	European Price
Zoloft®	100 50 mg	$80.00	$65.00
Pravachol®	28 10 mg	$55.60	$31.00

THERE IS A FREE-MARKET SOLUTION

We at Life Extension® have long espoused an easy solution to drug price gouging, which is to amend the Food, Drug, and Cosmetic Act to allow competition in the generic marketplace. If enacted, generic prices will plummet to levels so low you won't even worry about what percentage your insurance company pays. When generic drugs drop this much, it will push down many patented pharmaceutical prices because generic substitutes often work as well as newer branded drugs.

Against us are pharmaceutical lobbyists who will do virtually anything to protect their lucrative monopoly against free-market competition. On our side are 330 million American consumers, most of whom cannot afford to fall ill even if they have health insurance. That's because the deductibles, co-pays, and exclusions result in enormous out-of-pocket expenses that are today's leading cause of personal bankruptcies.

FIGHT BACK AGAINST FDA TYRANNY!

In 1992, the FDA proposed to re-classify certain dietary supplements as prescription drugs. This ignited an avalanche of protests by consumers.

Congress was inundated with letters demanding legislation to prevent the FDA from censoring access to natural ingredients that had demonstrated health benefits. The result was passage of the Dietary Supplement Health and

Education Act in 1994.[12] This Act spared many lives by providing consumers with affordable access to nutrients like coenzyme Q10 and higher-potency vitamin D.

Life Extension® continues to coordinate with other health freedom groups to stop Big Pharma from further monopolizing consumer access to effective conventional medical care. We need the support of readers of this book to win these battles.

For those who think it's not worth the effort, consider the consequences of failing to take action.

Innovation in the natural ingredient marketplace will be stifled while pharmaceutical companies take the same ingredients and gain FDA protection to sell them as prescription drugs. Many retired seniors will have to take jobs to afford their medications. Those working full time may have to find additional part-time work to pay the high premiums and many out-of-pocket expenses no longer covered by medical insurance. These problems can be partially resolved if free-market competition is allowed in the generic drug and dietary supplement marketplaces.

LOG ON TO OUR LEGISLATIVE ACTION WEBSITE

Life Extension® has ongoing grassroots campaigns to overwhelm lobbyists that dominate Congress and federal agencies. We maintain a website with the current Representatives and Senators so you can easily send emails protesting legislation that restricts competition, stifles biomedical innovation and unnecessarily drives up drug prices.

To let your voice be heard on Capitol Hill please log on to: StopFDA.org

References

1. Life Extension Wins in the House and Senate. Available at: http://www.stopfda.org/sep2000_awsi.htm. Accessed Oct. 27, 2016.

2. New England Journal of Medicine Exposes Generic Price Scandal. Available at: http://www.lifeextension.com/Magazine/2016/3/New-England-Journal-of-Medicine-Exposes-Generic-Price-Scandal/Page-01. Accessed Oct. 27, 2016.

3. Burden of Health-Care Costs Moves to the Middle Class. Available at: http://liveclinic.com/blog/healthcare-news/burden-u-s-health-care-costs-moving-middle-class/. Accessed Oct. 27, 2016.

4. Under Pressure: Shifts in Household Spending Over the Past 30 Years. Available at: https://www.brookings.edu/blog/up-front/2016/06/03/under-pressure-shifts-in-household-spending-over-the-past-30-years/. Accessed Oct. 28, 2016.

5. 2016 Employer Health Benefits Survey. Available at: http://kff.org/report-section/ehbs-2016-summary-of-findings/. Accessed Oct. 28, 2016.

6. Payments for Cost Sharing Increasing Rapidly Over Time. Available at: http://kff.org/health-costs/issue-brief/payments-for-cost-sharing-increasing-rapidly-over-time/. Accessed Oct. 28, 2016.

7. The price of an EpiPen has skyrocketed more than 500% since 2009 — and senators are asking for answers. Available at: http://www.businessinsider.com/epipen-price-increases-about-500-percent-2016-8. Accessed Nov. 1, 2016.

8. People are furious about the price of the EpiPen — here's how much it's increased in the last decade. Available at: http://www.businessinsider.com/how-much-price-of-mylans-epipen-has-increased-2016-8. Accessed Nov. 1, 2016.

9. It's Jaw-Dropping How Little It Costs to Make an EpiPen. Available at: http://time.com/money/4481786/how-much-epipen-costs-to-make/. Accessed Nov. 1, 2016.

10. The $300 generic EpiPen from Mylan shows drug pricing is broken in the United States. Available at: https://mic.com/articles/152912/generic-epipen-mylan-half-price-300-dollars-still-shows-drug-pricing-crisis-in-the-united-states#. U1vUJo97O. Accessed Nov. 2, 2016.

11. How Obama's FDA Keeps Generic Drugs off the Market. Available at: http://www.wsj.com/articles/how-obamas-fda-keeps-generic-drugs-off-the-market-1471645550. Accessed Nov. 2, 2016.

12. Dietary Supplement Health and Education Act of 1994. Availableat:https://www.congress.gov/bill/103rd-congress/senate-bill/784.

Epilogue

A S I WAS CONCLUDING THIS BOOK, some interesting developments were occurring that corroborate what you've read up until now. I summarize these in this concluding epilogue:

BRAND-NAME DRUG PRICES RISE AT SHOCKING RATE

A study published in the final days of 2016 found that older Americans are being gouged by the prices of brand-name drugs, which skyrocketed last year at a rate 130 times faster than inflation.*

Researchers at the nonprofit organization AARP discovered that the retail prices of 268 brand-name prescription drugs rose, on average, 15.5% in 2015 against a 0.1% increase in the rate of general inflation. The drugs, which are commonly taken by seniors, include 49 that are used to treat diabetes, high cholesterol, high blood pressure and other wide-spread, chronic conditions.

Debra Whitman, chief public policy officer at AARP, stated in a news release, "What's particularly remarkable is

---

* Available at: http://tinyurl.com/jpr8p5q. Accessed December 15, 2016.

that these incredibly high price increases are still occurring in the face of intense public and congressional criticism of prescription drug pricing practices."

"Prescription drug therapy is not affordable when its cost exceeds the patient's entire income," said report co-author Leigh Purvis. "Even if patients are fortunate enough to have good healthcare coverage, high prescription drug costs translate into higher out-of-pocket costs."

EDITOR'S NOTE: According to the study, of the six drugs with the highest price increases, five were from Valeant Pharmaceuticals. The study's authors found the price of Ativan®, the company's antianxiety drug, shot up over 2,800% between 2006 and 2015. The cost of the active ingredient in this drug is virtually nothing, but the price nonetheless spiraled upwards. If you wonder how this can happen, a simpler answer may be price-fixing among generic makers. This situation could not occur if there was a real free market when it comes to generic drug manufacture and sale. Instead, all generic drug makers need the FDA's blessing before selling an off-patent drug that is no more complex to manufacture than a dietary supplement.

FORMER DRUG COMPANY EXECS CHARGED IN PRICE-FIXING PLOT

As part of an ongoing Department of Justice investigation into the generic drug industry, charges have been brought against two ex-drug company executives for allegedly participating in a bid-rigging and price-fixing plot.*

Named in separate two-count felony cases were Jason Malek, the former president of Heritage Pharmaceuticals, and Jeffrey Glazer, the company's former CEO. The alleged

---

* Available at: http://tinyurl.com/z9rl3yo. Accessed December 15, 2016.

scheme involved two drugs: the diabetes medication glyburide and doxycycline hyclate, an antibiotic. According to court papers filed in Philadelphia, the scheme was in effect possibly dating back to April 2013 and continued to December 2015.

The cost of 500 tablets of doxycycline is reported to have gone from $20 in October 2013 to a whopping $1,845 in May 2014.

Deputy Assistant Attorney General Brent Snyder charged that the two executives entered into unlawful agreements to fix prices and "sought to enrich themselves at the expense of sick and vulnerable individuals who rely upon access to generic pharmaceuticals as a more affordable alternative to brand-name medicines."

Following an internal investigation, Heritage had fired both men. Reacting to the charges, the company stated the former executives had engaged in "a variety of serious misconduct."

EDITOR'S NOTE: In a prepared statement, Special Agent in Charge Michael Harpster of the FBI's Philadelphia division commented, "Conspiring to fix prices on widely-used generic medications skews the market, flouts common decency, and very clearly breaks the law. It's a sad state of affairs when these pharmaceutical executives are determined to further pad their profits on the backs of people whose health depends on the company's drugs."

If any or all of the documented atrocities revealed in this book are of concern to you, then please let your voice be heard on Capitol Hill. You can conveniently do this by logging on to www.STOPFDA.org.

Index

G